Articles on stand
Milliamperes
Contents of Case - (silk, bandage, ____ dressings)
Contents of Desk - band inst.__ ____ medicine ca
Medicine on desk
McCune chisels
Small chisels

To Dr₂

TELEPHONE 1512.
OFFICE OPEN AT ALL HOURS.

____rs

To Professional Services Render___

____rile, Dr.   1 Clamp

                                           50
                                      1   00
                    1411 | 75   ____ 50 $ 1778 | 10
                       2 | 00
                       2 | 00
                       5 | 00
                       2 | 00

Cleveland O. Apr 10th 1891.
____ation of seventeen hundred
____ ____ dollars I ____ hereby this
____rs F. E. Bunts and G. W. Crile
____ Chattels, Instruments and other
____ in brick house and
at No 380 Pearl St
____ory marked exhibit "A" attached
____.
                    C H Wood
                    Administrator of Frank J Wie___

"…to act as a unit"

THE STORY
OF THE
CLEVELAND CLINIC

Contributors

F. Merlin Bumpus, M.D.

George Crile, Jr., M.D.

Victor G. deWolfe, M.D.

Mary Rita Feran, M.S.

Stanley O. Hoerr, M.D.

Carol M. Tomer, M.S.

William S. Kiser, M.D.

Fay A. Le Fevre, M.D.

William M. Michener, M.D.

William L. Proudfit, M.D.

"…to act as a unit"

The Story
of the
Cleveland Clinic

Shattuck W. Hartwell, Jr., M.D., editor

1985
W. B. Saunders Company
Philadelphia London Toronto Mexico City Rio de Janeiro Sydney Tokyo

W. B. Saunders Company: West Washington Square
Philadelphia, PA 19105

1 St. Anne's Road
Eastbourne, East Sussex BN21 3UN, England

1 Goldthorne Avenue
Toronto, Ontario M8Z 5T9, Canada

Apartado 26370   Cedro 512
Mexico 4, D.F., Mexico

Rua Coronel Cabrita, 8
Sao Cristovao Caixa Postal 21176
Rio de Janeiro, Brazil

9 Waltham Street
Artarmon, N.S.W. 2064, Australia

Ichibancho, Central Bldg., 22–1 Ichibancho
Chiyoda-Ku, Tokyo 102, Japan

Library of Congress Cataloging in Publication Data

Main entry under title:

To act as a unit.

  Bibliography: p.
  Includes index.
  1. Cleveland Clinic—History. 2. Clinics—Ohio—
Cleveland—History. I. Hartwell, Shattuck W.
(Shattuck Wellman), 1928–   II. Bumpus, F. Merlin.
[DNLM: 1. Cleveland Clinic. 2. Ambulatory Care
Facilities—history—Ohio. WX 28 A03 C6C6t]
RA982.C62C558   1985   362.1'1'0977131   84-24049
ISBN 0-7216-1709-3

". . .to act as a unit": The Story of the Cleveland Clinic   ISBN   0–7216–1709–3

Last digit is the print number: 9   8   7   6   5   4   3   2   1

To the Memory of the Founders

FRANK E. BUNTS, 1861–1928

GEORGE W. CRILE, 1864–1943

WILLIAM E. LOWER, 1867–1948

JOHN PHILLIPS, 1879–1929

CONTENTS

ILLUSTRATIONS   ix

PREFACE   xi

FOREWORD   xiii

ONE
THE FOUNDERS.   1

TWO
THE FIRST YEARS, 1921–1929   13

THREE
THE DISASTER, 1929   25

FOUR
THE PHOENIX, 1929–1941   33

FIVE
TURBULENT SUCCESS, 1941–1955   39

SIX
TRUSTEES AND GOVERNORS, 1955–1984.   49
Issues of Management, Growth, and Control   49

SEVEN
". . . BETTER CARE OF THE SICK"   67
Division of Medicine.   67
Division of Surgery   82
Division of Anesthesiology   104
Division of Radiology   107

Division of Laboratory Medicine 114

EIGHT
". . . INVESTIGATION OF THEIR PROBLEMS" 123
Division of Research 123

NINE
". . . FURTHER EDUCATION OF THOSE WHO SERVE." 133
Division of Education 133

NOTES 139

INDEX.. 172

ILLUSTRATIONS

FRONTISPIECE   The Founders

Offices at 16 Church Street 2
Offices at 380 Pearl Street 6
Osborn Building at East 9th and Huron 7
Bunts and Crile, 1918 9
Clinic Building, 1921 15
Waiting Room, 1921... 15
Oxley Homes, 1924 22
Cleveland Clinic Hospital, 1930s 22
The Disaster, May 15, 1929 28
Cleveland Clinic, East 93rd Street, 1935 35
Henry S. Sherman 38
Edward C. Daoust 41
John Sherwin 42
Clarence M. Taylor 44
Board of Governors, 1956....................................... 50
Fay A. LeFevre, M.D. 51
Carl E. Wasmuth, M.D. 56
Cleveland Clinic, Aerial View, 1969 56
Harry T. Marks, William S. Kiser, M.D., James A. Hughes 61
New Clinic, 1985 64
New Hospital, 1985 64
Russell L. Haden, M.D. 68
Thomas E. Jones, M.D. 86
Robert S. Dinsmore, M.D.. 88
Cardiac Team, 1956 101
René G. Favaloro, M.D., and F. Mason Sones, Jr., M.D........... 102
Otto Glasser, Ph.D. 109
Meyer Medical Magnetic Resonance Center, 1983 111
John Beach Hazard, M.D. 115
Laboratory Medicine Building, 1980 119

ix

Irvine H. Page, M.D. 125
Research Building, 1974 132
Education Building, 1964 137

PREFACE

In 1981 the Board of Governors of The Cleveland Clinic Foundation authorized the publication of a second edition of *TO ACT AS A UNIT*. The first edition published in 1971 was a chronicle of the institution's first half century. In the 13 years since the first edition, growth and changes in the practice of medicine have made the Clinic a different institution from what it had been in the first fifty years. A new book was needed to tell that part of the story.

This edition draws heavily on the first, even though much has been rewritten. Chapters One through Four contain material compiled by the late Dr. Alexander T. Bunts and Dr. George Crile, Jr. Dr. William L. Proudfit wrote Chapter Seven, Dr. F. Merlin Bumpus wrote Chapter Eight, and Dr. William M. Michener wrote Chapter Nine. These chapters comprise the histories of the five Divisions of Clinical Practice and the Divisions of Research and Education.

Conserving essential information and updating the material from the first edition, Dr. Stanley O. Hoerr has written Chapter Five. I have rewritten the history of the Board of Governors, Chapter Six.

Contributors to the first edition were Dr. Alexander T. Bunts, Dr. George Crile, Jr., Dr. A. Carlton Ernstene, Mr. James G. Harding, Dr. John Beach Hazard, Dr. C. Robert Hughes, Dr. Fay A. LeFevre, Dr. Irvine H. Page, Mr. John Sherwin, Dr. Carl E. Wasmuth, and Dr. Walter J. Zeiter. Their names appeared on the title page of that book. Drs. Bunts, Ernstene, Hughes, and LeFevre have since died. The names of the contributors to this edition appear on the title page. They functioned as a committee, meeting many many times. I was asked to be their Chairman, and so befell to me the task of collecting, organizing, and editing all of the material that composes this book. I have enjoyed this assignment. The generous commitment of time and talent given to me by each member of the committee is gratefully acknowledged.

I must give special thanks to Diane L. Crouse, Mary Rita Feran, and Carol M. Tomer. Ms. Crouse painstakingly prepared every draft of the book. I depended heavily on Miss Feran's editorial skill in matters of style and usage. Mrs. Tomer, Archivist of The Cleveland Clinic Foundation, was tireless in tending to the countless details that are essential to the successful completion of any important task.

SHATTUCK W. HARTWELL, JR., M.D., EDITOR
Cleveland, Ohio
March 1984

FOREWORD

The Cleveland Clinic Foundation was incorporated in 1921 as an alternative to the office practice of individual physicians and surgeons of that era. The founders believed that medical practice and teaching and research could be improved by the collaboration of physicians and scientists working together in one organization. Thus began an institution that was to become one of the world's great centers of medicine.

A tragic disaster costing many lives, the grinding hardships of the great depression, and the troublesome quest for secure leadership were tests of survival in the first thirty years. Tempered by these challenges, the Clinic entered the second half of the twentieth century with confidence. The members of the professional staff have a reputation for excellence in treatment of complex medical problems and in the past three decades an increasing number of patients have been attracted from throughout the world.

As this phase of history is documented, The Cleveland Clinic Foundation, like all other health care institutions throughout the nation, faces an uncertain future. In America there are now tumultuous changes that are reshaping the health care system. The escalating cost of health care, resulting largely from the Federal programs that made American medicine the best in the world, has led to a national crisis. Reactive and radical restructuring of reimbursement mechanisms that limit payment to hospitals and doctors has promoted intense competition among providers of health care. Determined to remain a leader, the Cleveland Clinic is responding to the economic mandate by expansion of services and innovative changes in organizational structure. Perhaps The Cleveland Clinic Foundation of the future will be a comprehensive health care delivery system, even international in scope, with activities of the Clinic integrated with services provided by physicians in other group practices of this region or throughout the country. Whatever is to be, the members of the professional staff of The Cleveland Clinic Foundation face the future with optimism and with an undiminished commitment to excellence in health care through group effort.

WILLIAM S. KISER, M.D.
Chairman, Board of Governors

xiii

The Founders

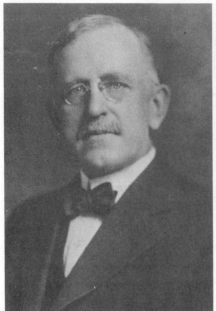

Dr. Frank E. Bunts

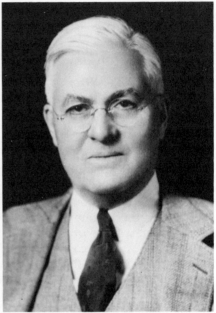

Dr. George W. Crile

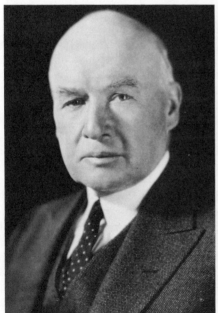

Dr. William E. Lower

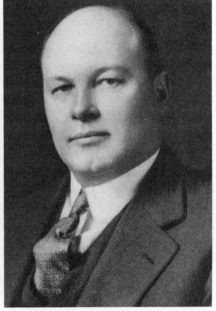

Dr. John Phillips

ONE

∎ THE FOUNDERS

On August 27, 1918, Dr. George W. Crile, who at the time was with the Lakeside Hospital Unit in France, wrote in his journal:

"What a remarkable record Bunts, Crile and Lower have had all these years. We have been rivals in everything, yet through all the vicissitudes of personal, financial and professional relations we have been able to think and act as a unit."[1]

This feeling of cooperation and unity, shared by three founders of the Cleveland Clinic, made it possible for the institution to be born.

Dr. Frank E. Bunts was the senior member of the three surgeons who had been so closely associated for many years before the founding of the Cleveland Clinic. After a brief career in the Navy, he attended medical school for three years at Western Reserve University and graduated in 1886 as valedictorian of his class. After a year of internship at St. Vincent Charity Hospital in Cleveland, he entered the office of Dr. Frank J. Weed, then Dean and Professor of Surgery at the Wooster University Department of Medicine, Cleveland, Ohio.

Dr. George W. Crile was born on a farm in Chili, Ohio, and he worked his way through Northwestern Ohio Normal School (later known as Ohio Northern University) in Ada by teaching in elementary schools. After receiving a teaching certificate, he was appointed Principal of the Plainfield (Ohio) School. Soon his interest was attracted to medicine, mainly as a result of his contacts with a local physician who loaned him books and with whom he visited patients. Some of the events of this period are related in his autobiography, among them exciting details of "quilling" an obstetric patient by blowing snuff through a goose quill into her nose. The

1

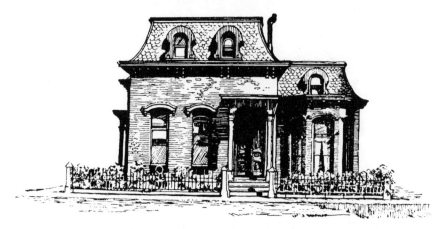

Offices of Drs. Weed, Bunts and Crile at 16 Church Street, 1886–1889
(artist's drawing)

sneezing that this induced led to prompt delivery of the baby. In 1886, Crile went to Wooster and after two years obtained his M.D. degree with highest honors.

Crile served his internship at University Hospital under Dr. Frank J. Weed,[2] and after that he joined Bunts as an assistant to Weed in his large office practice. Then, at age 45 and at the peak of his professional career, Weed contracted pneumonia and died. At that time, Bunts was not yet 30 years old and Crile was three years younger. Crile expressed their feelings as follows:

"Wearied by loss of sleep, worry and constant vigil, we left Doctor Weed's house on that cheerless March morning and walked to Doctor Bunts's for breakfast. In our dejection, it seemed to us that everything had suddenly come to an end. Our light had gone out. We had no money, no books, no surgical instruments. The only instrument either of us owned, other than my microscope, was a stethoscope. But we agreed to carry on together, to share and share alike both the expenses and the income from the accident practice, each to reserve for himself the income from his private patients."

After talking with Mrs. Weed, Bunts and Crile decided to buy, from the estate, Dr. Weed's goods, chattels and instruments. Excerpts from the Bill of Sale are listed below.[3] This property represented the embryo from which the Cleveland Clinic was born.

Bill of Sale
From Estate of Dr. Frank J. Weed
to
Dr. Frank E. Bunts and Dr. George Crile

Small brown mares (Brown Jug and Roseline)	$125.00
Small sorrel horse (Duke).............................	100.00
Bay horse (Roy)	75.00
Top buggy	50.00
Top buggy	50.00
Top buggy, very old	10.00
Open buggy	20.00
2 Cutters—one very old	20.00
4 Sets single harness.................................	20.00
Lap robes	15.00
Miscellaneous articles in barn	3.00
Shed, old stoves, battery, etc........................	50.00

••••••••

Articles on stand	20.00
Milliamperes	10.00
Contents of Case—(silk, bandages and dressings).......	15.00
Contents of Desk—hand mirror, 6 sprinklers, medicine case	8.00
Medicine on desk....................................	25.00
3 McCune chisels	3.75
4 Small chisels.......................................	2.00
14 Pairs scissors	2.50
3 Large pairs shears.................................	1.50
2 Pairs retractors....................................	2.00
2 Forceps	2.50
3 Nasal saws	1.50
2 Intestinal clasps...................................	1.00
1 Chain saw...	2.00
2 Hayes saws	1.50
1 Small met. saw	.50
7 Needles	1.00
4 Wire twisters	1.00
6 Sponge holders	1.50
1 Clamp	2.00

3 Bullet forceps 2.00
2 Large retractors 2.00
4 Small nasal dilators 1.25
1 Throat forcep 1.50
1 Head reflector 2.50
4 Self retaining female catheters.................. 1.75
2 Tools .... .50
5 Bone elevators 2.00
5 Bone forceps 6.00
1 Chain saw guide .... .75
1 Bone drill with three tips .... .75
1 Hamilton bone drill with four tips 3.00

•••••••

1 Emergency bag No. 2 .... 5.00
1 Emergency bag No. 3 .... 11.00
1 Box—3 knives and 3 pairs scissors 1.50
1 Stomach pump in box 6.00
1 Stone set in case 8.00
1 Horse shoe turnica 1.00
1 Cloven clutch 4.00
1 Small aspirating set 2.00
1 Kelley pad .... .75
1 Syringe .... .50
1 Microscope 40.00
2 Syringes 1.50

Total $1778.10

Cleveland, O., Apr. 10th, 1891

In consideration of seventeen hundred and seventy eight 10/100 dollars I have this day sold to Drs. F.E. Bunts and G.W. Crile all the goods, chattels, instruments and other articles contained in brick house and barn in rear at No. 380 Pearl Street as per inventory marked Exhibit A attached to bill of sale.

C. H. Weed,
Administrator of Frank J. Weed

The practice of the new partners increased rapidly, with the result that in 1892 an associate was needed. Dr. William E. Lower, a cousin of Crile, was engaged; both had attended district schools. Lower, too, had been reared on a farm and from an early age had to look out for himself, learning the meaning of hard work and the necessity of thrift and frugality, traits that were to remain an integral part of his character. Lower had attended the Medical Department of Wooster University, from which he was graduated in 1891; he served as house physician in City Hospital, and then set up practice in Conneaut, Ohio. Bunts and Crile had little difficulty in persuading him to leave there and to share their office practice. This was the beginning of the "triple alliance," which was to continue throughout their lives. By 1895, Bunts, Crile, and Lower were full partners, each sharing equally the expenses and the income from emergency work, but remaining competitors in private practice. Mutual trust and confidence became a keystone for their future accomplishments.

As their practice grew, Bunts, Crile, and Lower moved their office in 1897 from the west side of Cleveland downtown to the Osborn Building, at the junction of Huron Road and Prospect Avenue. A year later, practice was interrupted by the Spanish-American War; Bunts was surgeon to the First Ohio Volunteer Cavalry Unit of the Ohio National Guard, and Crile was surgeon to the Gatling Gun Battery in Cleveland, also a unit of the Guard. When they volunteered for active duty, Lower was left alone with the office practice. Not long after the war was over and his partners had returned, he retaliated by volunteering to help quell the Boxer Rebellion in China, entering the Army as a first lieutenant. By the time he reached China the rebellion was over, so he served as surgeon to the 9th U.S. Cavalry in the Philippines, 1900–1901.

By 1901 the various wars were over, and Bunts, Crile, and Lower were reunited in the Osborn Building office, where they remained until separated again by World War I. The prewar period was a productive one. In addition to their large accident and private practices, Bunts became professor of principles of surgery at Wooster University and professor of principles of surgery and clinical surgery at the Western Reserve University School of Medicine. Crile was professor of physiology and principles of surgery at Wooster and professor of surgery at Western Reserve. Lower, whose major interest soon became urology, was associate professor of genito-urinary surgery at Western Reserve.

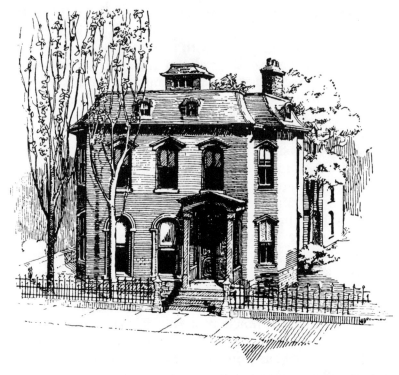

Offices of Drs. Bunts, Crile and Lower at 380 Pearl Street (now West 25th Street), 1890–1897   (artist's drawing)

During these years, Crile maintained his interest in physiology and applied to clinical practice the principles that he discovered in the laboratory in the fields of shock, transfusion, and anesthesia. Lower collaborated in some of Crile's early works, but neither he nor Bunts shared Crile's consuming and lifelong interest in basic laboratory research.

As the practice expanded, Dr. H. G. Sloan, a surgeon, was added to the staff, and Dr. J. D. Osmond was sent to the Mayo Clinic to observe the newly developed technics of radiology. Osmond returned to establish, in 1913, the group's first X-Ray Department. Dr. T. P. Shupe also joined the staff as an associate of Lower in urology.

During the period in which the Bunts, Crile, and Lower group was expanding, Crile was helping to mastermind the founding of The American College of Surgeons, whose purposes and functions

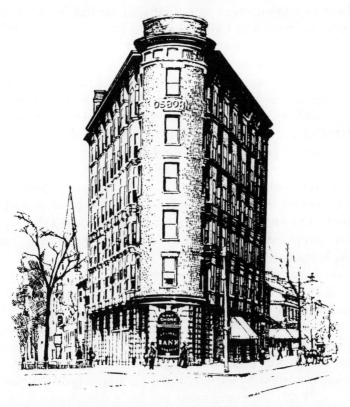

Offices of Drs. Bunts, Crile and Lower, Osborn Building at East 9th Street and Huron Road, 1897–1920   (artist's drawing)

were to improve the standards of surgical practice in the United States and Canada and to provide postgraduate education, to improve ethics, to raise the standards of care in hospitals, and to educate the public about medical and surgical problems. Travel from coast to coast to the many meetings of the College was time-consuming in those days before jet aircraft.

In 1914 Europe was ablaze in war. In December of that year, Crile, who was then Chief Surgeon at Lakeside Hospital, was asked by Clevelander Myron T. Herrick, then Ambassador to Paris, to organize a team to work in France. Crile accepted, for even at that time it seemed to him that the United States would be drawn into the war and that experience in military surgery would be valuable.[4]

After three months of treating casualties near the front, at Neuilly, the group returned, and Crile organized a base-hospital unit.

When the United States entered the war, the Lakeside Unit, U.S. Army Base Hospital No. 4, was the first detachment of the American Expeditionary Forces to arrive in France, taking over a British General Hospital in Rouen on May 25, 1917. Crile was the hospital's Clinical Director, but later was given a broader assignment as Director of the Division of Research for the American Expeditionary Forces, a post that permitted him to move about and visit the stations wherever the action was.

Lower was with Crile in the Lakeside Unit, and soon Bunts, a reservist, was ordered to Camp Travis, Texas, leaving only Sloan and Osmond to keep the practice going. Both were able to pay the office expenses, but Bunts, concerned about the future, wrote to Lower in France as follows:

"I feel very strongly that we ought to hold the office together at all hazards, not only for ourselves, but for the younger men who have been with us and whose future will depend largely on having a place to come back to. If Sloan and Osmond go, I think we could at least keep Miss Slattery and Miss Van Spyker. It would be quite an outlay for each of us to ante up our share for keeping the offices from being occupied by others, but I for one would be glad to do it. We haven't so very many years left for active work after this war is over, and it would seem to be almost too much to undertake to start afresh in new offices, and the stimulus and friendship of our old associations mean much more than money to me."

Bunts succeeded Lower as commanding officer of the hospital in Rouen in August 1918. After the armistice, November 11, 1918, activities at the Base Hospital gradually subsided, tension was eased, and soldiers found time to engage in nonmilitary pursuits and conversations. The long and friendly association of the three Cleveland surgeons is made clear from the following letter written in December 1918 and addressed to Lower in Cleveland from Bunts in France.

"It's getting around Christmas time, and while I know this won't reach you for a month, yet I just want to let you know that we are thinking of you and wishing we could see you. Crile has been here for a couple of weeks, but left again for Paris a few days ago, and evenings he and I have foregathered about the little stove in your old room, leaving G. W.'s door open wide enough to warm

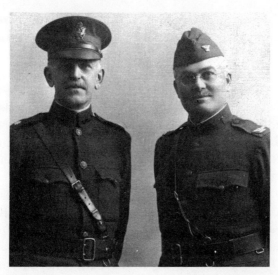

Lt. Col. Frank E. Bunts and Col. George W. Crile at Rouen, France, 1918

his room up too, and there we have sat like two old G.A.R. relics, smoking and laughing, telling stories, dipping back into even our boyhood days and laughing often till the tears rolled down our cheeks. It has been a varied life we three have had and filled with trials and pleasures without number. I have dubbed our little fireside chats the 'Arabian Nights,' and often we have been startled when the coal gave out and the fire died down that it was long past midnight and time for antiques to go to bed."

During those nocturnal chats at Rouen an idea was born that led to the founding of The Cleveland Clinic Foundation. The experience in a military hospital impressed these men with the efficiency of an organization that included every branch or specialty of medicine and surgery. They gained insight into the benefits that could be obtained when a group of specialists cooperated. Before their return to the United States they began to formulate plans for the future.

Bunts and Crile returned to Cleveland early in 1919 and were once more united with Lower in their Osborn Building offices. They began to recover their surgical practices that had been interrupted for two years and soon found themselves as busy as they had been before the war.

Although the military hospital was used as a model for their future plan, elements of the pattern were furnished also by the Mayo Clinic, founded by close professional friends. Bunts, Crile, and Lower were surgeons, and in order to develop a broader field of medical service they resolved to add an internist to organize and head a department of medicine. They were fortunate to obtain the enthusiastic cooperation of Dr. John Phillips, who was at that time a member of the faculty of the School of Medicine of Western Reserve University. He, too, had served in military hospitals during the war and held the same broad concept of what might be accomplished by a clinic organization.

John Phillips was born in 1879 on a farm near Welland, Ontario, and was said to have been a quiet, serious-minded youth who nevertheless had a keen sense of humor. After qualifying for a teacher's certificate, he taught for three years in a district school. He then entered the Faculty of Medicine in the University of Toronto, where in 1903 he received the M.B. degree with honors. After graduation he served for three years as intern and resident in medicine at Lakeside Hospital in Cleveland. He then entered practice as an associate in the office of Dr. E. F. Cushing, professor of pediatrics at Western Reserve. During the years before the founding of the Cleveland Clinic, Phillips served on the staff of the School of Medicine of Western Reserve University as assistant professor of medicine and assistant professor of therapeutics. Simultaneously he held hospital appointments at Babies' Dispensary and Hospital and at Lakeside Hospital. He was also consulting physician to St. John Hospital. Phillips had a large private and consulting practice and was highly regarded for his ability as clinician and teacher in the fields of internal medicine and the diseases of children. During the war he had served as a captain in the Medical Corps of the United States Army.

In 1920, group practice was by no means popular with private physicians, some of whom felt that the large resources available in a group clinic might give them unfair competition. Many were openly critical of the idea and might have attempted to block it had not the position of the founders in the medical community been unassailable. All of them were professors in one or more of the Cleveland medical schools. Crile was a major national and international figure in surgery and in national medical organizations; Lower was already well known nationally as a urologic surgeon; Phillips had a solid reputation locally and nationally in internal medicine; and Bunts's professional and personal reputation was of the highest order.

The reputation of the founders was not focused solely in the medical schools; it also was well established in the community hospitals. They held appointments at Cleveland General, University, City, St. Alexis, St. Vincent Charity, Lutheran, St. John, Lakeside, and Mount Sinai hospitals. Moreover, many of the business leaders of the community were their patients and friends. It would have been difficult to stand in the way of any legitimate enterprise that these physicians decided to organize. Perhaps this point could be emphasized by a thumbnail sketch of the personality of each, as Dr. George Crile, Jr., remembers them.

"Crile was the dynamo of the group, imaginative, creative, innovative, and driving. It is possible that some considered him inconsiderate of others in his overriding desire to get things done. For this reason, and because he occasionally was premature in applying to the treatment of patients the principles learned in research, he had enemies as well as supporters. Yet most of his contemporaries would have readily admitted that Crile was one of the first surgeons in the world to apply physiologic research to surgical problems, that he was one of the country's leaders in organizing and promoting medical organizations such as The American College of Surgeons, of which he became the president, and that it was largely as a result of Crile's energy, prestige, and practice that the Cleveland Clinic was founded.

"If Crile was the driver, Lower was the brake. He was a born conservative, even to the point of the keyhole size of his surgical incisions. No one but he could operate through them. His assistants could not even see into them. He was a technician of consummate skill and an imaginative pioneer in the then new field of urology. Lower was also a perfect treasurer. He checked on every expenditure, thus compensating for Crile's tendency to disregard the Clinic's cash position. Later in life, Doctor Lower even went around the buildings, in the evenings, turning out lights that were burning needlessly. He was no miser, but his conservatism afforded a perfect balance to Crile's overenthusiasm. Despite the differences in their personalities, no one ever saw them quarrel.

"I never knew Bunts as well as the others, for he died early, but I do recall that he never, in my presence at least, displayed the exuberant type of humor that Crile and Lower did. I have seen the latter two almost rolling on the floor in laughter as they reminisced on how they dealt with some ancient enemy, but I could not imagine Bunts doing that. He had the presence and dignity that one associates with the image of an old-time senator. 'Bunts was invaluable in our association,' my father once told me. 'He was the one that gave it respectability.'

"Phillips, like Bunts, died early, so that I knew him only as my childhood physician rather than as a personal friend. My impression was of a man who was silent, confident, and imperturbable. I am sure that his patients and colleagues shared this confidence in him, and that was why he was able to organize a successful department of internal medicine.

"Although the personalities of the Clinic's founders were so different from one another, there were common bonds that united them. All had served in the military, all had taught in medical schools, all were devoted to the practice of medicine. As a result of these common backgrounds and motivations, there emerged a common ideal—an institution in which medicine and surgery could be practiced, studied, and taught by a group of associated specialists. To create it, the four founders began to plan an institution that would be greater than the sum of its individual parts."

TWO

■ THE FIRST YEARS
1921–1929

In October 1919, the founders, with the aid of Mr. Edward C. Daoust, an able attorney and the son-in-law of Bunts, formed the Association Building Company for the purpose of financing, erecting, and equipping the Clinic building. Organized as a corporation for profit, the company issued common and preferred stock, most of which was bought by the founders and their families. Land on the southwest corner of East 93rd Street and Euclid Avenue was purchased. The architectural firm of Ellerbe and Company estimated that a suitable building could be erected for $400,000. Excavation began in February 1920, and a year later the building was completed. Although the Crowell-Little Company were the contractors, Dr. Crile said in his autobiography that ". . . the real builder of the Clinic was Ed Lower, he knew each brick and screw by name and was on hand early enough every morning to check the laborers as they arrived."

The Clinic building had four stories, and the upper three were built around a large central well that extended from the second floor up to a skylight of tinted glass. The central or 'well' part of the second floor was the main waiting room, handsome with tiled floors and walls and with arched tiled doorways and windows. The offices, examining rooms, and treatment rooms in the various departments opened onto the corridors of the balconies that surrounded the central well on the second, third, and fourth floors. On the first floor of the building were the x-ray department, the clinical laboratories, and a pharmacy. On the fourth floor were the art and photographic departments, editorial offices, a library, a board room in which the founders met, offices for administration and bookkeeping, and Dr.

Crile's biophysics laboratory. Thus, from the beginning there were departments representing not only the cooperative practice of medicine, but also education and research.

From the time of the incorporation of The Cleveland Clinic Foundation as a corporation not for profit, there were no shareholders and no profits accrued to the founders. All of them received fixed salaries set by the trustees. All other members of the Clinic staff likewise received fixed salaries, not directly dependent on the amount of income that they brought into the Clinic. By Ohio statute, no part of the earnings can accrue to the benefit of private individuals.[1]

The founders had donated substantially to the Clinic's capital funds, and in the formative years they had taken the risk of underwriting personally the Clinic's debts in order to establish a non-profit foundation dedicated to service of the community, medical education, and research. Moreover, to insure against any future deviation from these aims, the founders gave power to the Board of Trustees, at their discretion, to give all assets of the Foundation to any local institution incorporated "for promoting education, science, or art." The assets of the Foundation could never become the personal enrichment of any person.

At the first meeting of the incorporators on February 21, 1921, the signers were elected Trustees of the Foundation, and provision was made for increasing the number of trustees to fifteen if it became desirable to do so. Bunts, Crile, Lower, and Phillips were designated Founders of the Foundation.

The Cleveland Clinic's charter is an extraordinary document for its time because the scope of medical practice defined therein was so liberal. The document also raised the issue of the corporate practice of medicine, much criticized at the time.

The practice of medicine in the United States had traditionally been founded on a doctor-patient relationship, in which an individual patient paid a fee for service to the doctor of his choice. The medical profession has always resisted attempts to change the basis of this relationship. Likewise, lawyers have wanted to preserve the lawyer-client relationship, threatened by large corporations, such as banks, that sought to sell legal services to customers through the offices of their salaried lawyers. If a corporation were allowed to do the same with the services of physicians, a precedent dangerous to

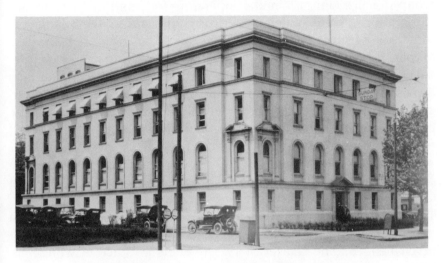

Clinic Building, 1921   The Cleveland Clinic Foundation

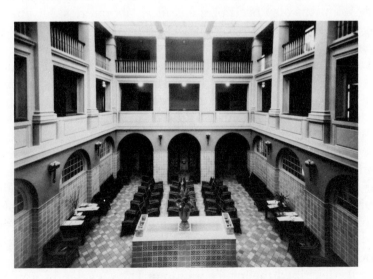

Waiting room, 1921   Clinic Building

the status of lawyers might be established. For this reason, most group-practice clinics, whether operating for profit or as nonprofit corporations, were obliged to incorporate within their structure some sort of professional partnership in order to bill patients and to collect fees legally. The properties of the Mayo Clinic, for example, have always been held by a nonprofit foundation. The physicians were organized first as a partnership and then as an association from 1919 to 1969. The doctors received salaries from the fees paid by patients and turned over to the Mayo Foundation the excess of receipts over disbursements.[2] Thus in most nonprofit clinics the same end has had to be attained by a devious route, which in the case of the Cleveland Clinic is accomplished directly; The Cleveland Clinic Foundation itself collects fees and pays the salaries of its staff. Today, with the strong trend toward group practice, the right of a nonprofit organization like the Clinic to "practice medicine" will not be challenged. The charter of 1921 remains a source of wonder to lawyers.

There were thirteen members of the professional staff of the Cleveland Clinic in its first year. Joining Bunts and Crile were Dr. Thomas E. Jones and Dr. Harry G. Sloan in surgery. Lower was joined by Dr. Thomas P. Shupe in urology. With Phillips in medicine were Dr. Henry J. John, Dr. Oliver P. Kimball, and Dr. John P. Tucker. Henry John was also head of the clinical laboratories. Dr. Justin M. Waugh was the otolaryngologist, Dr. Bernard H. Nichols was the radiologist, and Hugo Fricke, Ph.D. was in biophysics.

Crile was elected to be the first president of the Foundation; Bunts, vice president; Lower, treasurer; and Phillips, secretary. Daoust, who had so skillfully handled the Clinic's legal problems, was designated a life member of the Board of Trustees.

At 8:00 P.M. on February 26, 1921, five hundred local members of the medical profession and many physicians from out of the city attended the opening of the Cleveland Clinic. Among those from other cities were Dr. William J. Mayo of Rochester, Minnesota; Dr. Joseph C. Bloodgood of Baltimore, Maryland; and Dr. J. F. Baldwin of Columbus, Ohio. The program included talks by each of the founders and by president Charles Howe of Case School of Applied Science. Mayo gave the main address.

Crile described the incorporation of The Cleveland Clinic Foundation and outlined its purposes and aims as follows:

"With the rapid advance of medicine to its present-day status in which it evokes the aid of all the natural sciences, an individual is no more able to undertake the more intricate problems alone, without the aid and cooperation of colleagues having special training in each of the various clinical and laboratory branches, than he would be today to make an automobile alone. We have, therefore, created an organization and a building to the end that in making a diagnosis or planning a treatment, the clinician may have at his disposal the advantages of the laboratories of the applied sciences and of colleagues with special training in the various branches of medicine and surgery.

"Another reason for establishing this organization is that of making permanent our long-time practice of expending for research a goodly portion of our income. On this occasion we are pleased to state that we and our successors are pledged to give not less than one-fourth of our net income toward building up the property and the endowment of The Cleveland Clinic Foundation. It is through The Cleveland Clinic Foundation under a state charter that a continual policy of active investigation of disease will be assured. That is to say, we are considering not only our duty to the patient of today, but no less our duty to the patient of tomorrow.

"It is moreover our purpose, also, pursuant to our practice in the past, that by reason of the convenience of the plant, the diminished overhead expense, and the accumulation of funds in the Foundation, the patient with no means and the patient with moderate means may have at a cost he can afford, as complete an investigation as the patient with ample means.

"The fourth reason for the establishment of this Clinic is educational. We shall offer a limited number of fellowships to approved young physicians who have had at least one year of hospital training, thus supplementing the hospital and the medical school. In addition there will be established a schedule of daily conferences and lectures for our group and for others who may be interested.

"This organization makes it possible to pass on to our successors experience and methods and special technical achievements without a break of continuity.

"Since this organization functions as an institution, it has no intention either to compete with, nor to supplant the individual practitioner who is the backbone of the profession and carries on his shoulder the burden of the professional work of the community. We wish only to supplement, to aid, and to cooperate with him.

"Since this institution is not a school of medicine, it cannot, if it would, compete in any way with the University, but what it proposes to do is to offer a hearty cooperation in every way we can with the University.

"Our institution is designed to meet what we believe to be a public need in a more flexible organization than is possible for the University to attain, because the University as a teaching organization must of necessity be departmentalized. As compared with the University, this organization has the advantage of plasticity; as compared with the individual practitioner it has the advantage of equipment.

"The result of such an organization will be that the entire staff— the bacteriologist, the pathologist, the biochemist, the physicist, the physiologist, and radiologist, no less than the internist and the general surgeon—each, we hope and believe, will maintain the spirit of collective work, and each of us will accept as our reward for work done, his respective part in the contribution of the group, however small, to the comfort, and usefulness, and the prolongation of human life.

"Should the successors seek to convert it into an institution solely for profit or personal exploitations, or otherwise materially alter the purpose for which it was organized, the whole property shall be turned over to one of the institutions of learning or science of this city."

Bunts reviewed the development of the idea of organizing the Clinic, and outlined the founders' aims and hopes for the future. He said that the founders hoped, in time to come, when their associates took the places of their predecessors, that they would ". . . carry on the work to higher and better ends, aiding their fellow practitioners, caring for the sick, educating and training younger men in all the advances in medicine and surgery, and seeking always to attain the highest and noblest aspirations of their profession."

Phillips, in his remarks, made it clear that in establishing the Clinic the founders had no desire to compete with the family physician, but sought to make it a place to which the general practitioner might send patients for a diagnostic survey.

Lower explained the design of the building and its plan of construction which would ensure the highest efficiency to each department and thereby the most efficient operation of the Clinic as a whole, for the ultimate welfare of the patients.

The main address of the evening was entitled "The Medical Profession and the Public." Its contents were most significant at that time, and it holds many truths and ideas which are still worthy of consideration. Mayo spoke in part as follows:

"On every side we see the acceptance of an idea which is generally expressed by the loose term 'group medicine,' a term which fails in many respects to express conditions clearly. In my father's time, success in the professions was more or less dependent on convention, tradition, and impressive surroundings. The top hat and the double-breasted frock coat of the doctor, the wig and gown of the jurist, and the clerical garb of the ecclesiastic supplied the necessary stage scenery. The practitioner of medicine today may wear a business suit. The known facts in medicine are so comprehensive that the standing of the physician in his profession and in his community no longer depends on accessories.

"So tremendous has been the recent advance of medicine that no one man can understand more than a small fraction of it; thus, physicians have become more or less dependent on the skill, ability, and specialized training of other physicians for sufficient knowledge to care for the patient intelligently. An unconscious movement for cooperative medicine is seen in the intimate relation of the private physician to the public health service made possible by the establishment of laboratories by the state board of health and similar organizations. On every hand, even among laymen, we see this growing conception of the futility of the individual effort to encompass the necessary knowledge needed in treating the simplest and most common maladies because of the many complications which experience has shown are inherent possibilities of any disease."

Mayo went on to discuss some of the fundamental political and professional aspects of medical care and ended by stating:

". . . of each hundred dollars spent by our government during 1920, only one dollar went to public health, agriculture and education, just one percent for life, living conditions and national progress. . . . The striking feature of the medicine of the immediate future will be the development of medical cooperation, in which the state, the community and the physician must play a part.

". . . properly considered, group medicine is not a financial arrangement, except for minor details, but a scientific cooperation for the welfare of the sick.

". . . Medicine's place is fixed by its services to mankind; if we fail to measure up to our opportunity, it means state medicine, political control, mediocrity, and loss of professional ideals. The members of the medical fraternity must cooperate in this work, and they can do so without interfering with private professional practice. Such a community of interest will raise the general level of professional attainments. The internist, the surgeon, and the specialist may join with the physiologist, the pathologist and the laboratory workers to form the clinical group, which must also include men learned in the abstract sciences, such as biochemistry and physics. Union of all these forces will lengthen by many years the span of human life and as a byproduct will do much to improve professional ethics by overcoming some of the evils of competitive medicine."

With these instructive and challenging remarks, Mayo emphasized the fundamental aims of the founders of the Cleveland Clinic, which, from the time of its incorporation, have been: "better care of the sick, investigation of their problems, and further education of those who serve."[3]

On Sunday, February 27, 1921, the Clinic held open house for some fifteen hundred visitors. On the following day it was open to the public, and forty-two new patients registered.

The Clinic was so well accepted by the public that it soon became apparent to the founders that they needed a hospital adjacent to it, even though they continued to have hospital privileges at Lakeside, Charity, and Mount Sinai hospitals. Crile had agreed with the trustees of Lakeside that he would retire as professor of surgery at Western Reserve in 1924, and Dr. Lower had entered into a similar agreement with the trustees of Mount Sinai Hospital. A question arose whether or not the hospitals would continue to make available a sufficient number of beds to the staff of the new clinic.

To be frozen out of hospital beds was a real possibility, and the first stopgap arrangement that was made was the purchase of two old houses on East 93rd Street just north of Carnegie Avenue.[4] These were converted into a 53-bed hospital, the Oxley Homes, named for the competent English nurse, Mrs. Oxley, who was put in charge. Another house was used by Dr. Henry John to treat diabetes, not easy in those days, for insulin had just been discovered and patients' reactions to it were not yet well understood. A fourth house was used for physiotherapy, a fifth for serving luncheons to the medical staff.

At first, Oxley Homes was considered to be essentially a nursing home. Soon, however, an operating room was installed in which major operations were performed. This practice presented some difficulties, because there were no elevators in the buildings. Orderlies, nurses, and doctors had to carry the patients up and down the stairs of the old houses. In the meantime, plans had been made to build a modern 184-bed hospital; this was opened June 14, 1924, and Miss Charlotte E. Dunning was put in charge.[5] The seventh floor contained operating rooms, living quarters for several of the residents, and the pathology and clinical laboratories. Although there were now 237 beds available, including the Oxley Homes, the demand for beds could not be met. Two years later two floors of the Bolton Square Hotel, located one block west on Carnegie Avenue, were equipped for the care of 40 medical patients.

The experience of the Cleveland Clinic with hospital beds can be summarized in the phrase, too few and too late. By 1928, the shortage was again acute, and construction was started on an extension of the Hospital through to 93rd Street to provide a total of 275 beds exclusive of Oxley Homes and the hotel rooms. The increasing needs for supplementary services made it necessary to install a machine shop in a penthouse on the Clinic building, and to erect a power plant, laundry and ice plant. Parking of cars became more and more of a problem, necessitating buying and razing a number of nearby houses to provide space.[6] By 1928, the biophysics laboratory in the Clinic building became inadequate, because of the expansion of research, and to compensate for this a narrow eight-story research building was erected between the Hospital and the Clinic.

In that same year, Bunts, who had appeared to be in good health and had been carrying on his practice as usual, died suddenly of a heart attack, an event that saddened all who knew him.[7] At a memorial meeting, held in the auditorium of the Clinic to honor Bunts's memory, Dr. C. F. Thwing, president of Western Reserve University and a member of the Board of Trustees of The Cleveland Clinic Foundation, said in the course of his address that Bunts had always

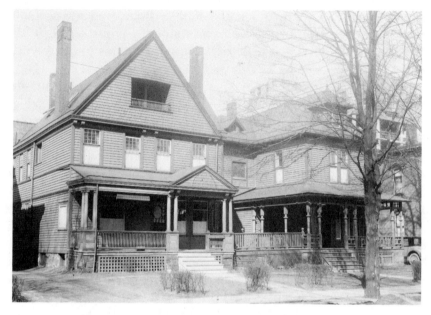

Oxley Homes, 1924

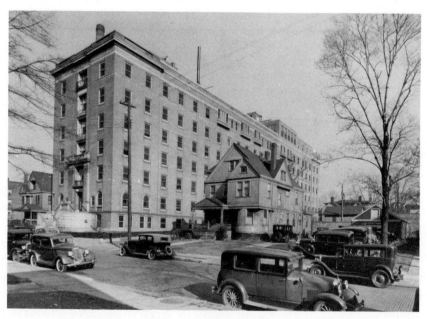

Cleveland Clinic Hospital, East 90th Street (photographed in the 1930s)

been ". . . responsive, heart to heart, mind to mind, and added to this responsiveness was a constant sense of restraint; he never overflowed; he never went too far. There was an old set of philosophers called the Peripatetics who were of this type. He held himself together. He was a being in whom integrity had unbounded rule and control."

Fortunately, the expanding work of the Clinic had led Bunts to appoint a young associate whom he had taught in medical school and in residency training and who now stood ready to take over Bunts's practice. This was Dr. Thomas E. Jones, who was destined to become one of the most brilliant technical surgeons of his time.

The number of patients registering at the Clinic and also the number of those requiring admission to the Hospital continued to rise steadily, so that to meet the demands the professional staff was increased and new departments were added. A gram of radium was donated to the Clinic by Mrs. James Packard, wife of the founder of the Packard Motor Company. A radium emanation plant, which made radon seeds to be used in the treatment of cancer, was installed in the therapy house, the first one in this part of the country. An x-ray therapy unit of the highest available quality also was installed, and Dr. U. V. Portmann, a highly trained specialist in radiation therapy, was put in charge. Portmann, in conjunction with Mr. Valentine Seitz, the brilliant engineer who was in charge of the machine shop, and Otto Glasser, Ph.D. of the Biophysics Department made the first dosimeter capable of measuring accurately the amount of radiation that was being given. Jones, now on the surgical staff, had had special training in the use of radium and radon seeds and was well prepared to take advantage of the new radiation facilities.

The Department of Radiotherapy was only one of the many new departments at the Cleveland Clinic. Medical specialties, such as endocrinology, were still in their infancy but growing fast. At the same time, surgery was becoming more and more specialized, requiring the addition of such departments as orthopedic surgery and neurological surgery. The Clinic was taking full advantage of the development of the specialties and of the prosperity that characterized the 1920s. It seemed that its spectacular growth would continue without interruption.

THREE

■ THE DISASTER
1929

On Wednesday, May 15, 1929, in the course of an otherwise normally busy working day at the Clinic, a calamity took place, resulting in great loss of life and threatening the future existence of the institution. Incomplete combustion of nitrocellulose x-ray films, which at that time were stored in a basement room of the Clinic Building, caused formation of vast quantities of toxic fumes and carbon monoxide. At least two explosions followed; toxic gases permeated the entire building and caused the deaths of 123 persons and the temporary illness of about 50.

The disaster occurred about 11:30 A.M. when there were about 250 patients, visitors, and employees in the Clinic Building. Fire did not present a major problem, because the building was fireproof. The damage to persons resulted from inhalation of toxic gases. The occupants of the nearby research building and hospital experienced no trouble whatever. Because a fire door closed the underground tunnel connecting these buildings, gas was confined to the Clinic.

The room in which old films were stored was located on the west side of the basement adjoining the rear elevator shaft. There was direct communication between this room and a horizontal pipe tunnel or chase, which made a complete circuit of the basement and from which nineteen vertical pipe ducts extended through partitions to the roof space. These provided the principal routes for the passage of gases throughout the building.

Old nitrocellulose x-ray films in manila envelopes, about three films to the envelope, were stored on wooden shelves and in standard steel files. The number of films in the room was not known, but it was estimated that there were about 70,000 or 4,200 pounds of

25

films of all sizes. Some estimates were as high as 10,000 pounds. Water pipes and three steam lines were located below the ceiling of the room. The steam lines were covered with insulation. One high-pressure steam line carrying about 65 pounds passed within seven and one-half inches of the nearest film shelf. The room had no outside ventilation. Light wiring was in conduit, with several pendant lamps. There were no automatic sprinklers.

Several hours before the disaster, a leak had been discovered in the high-pressure steam line in the film storage room. A steam fitter, who was called to make repairs, arrived about 9:00 A.M. and removed about fourteen inches of insulation allowing a jet of steam about three feet long to issue from the pipe in the direction of the film rack against the north wall. He went to the power house to close the steam line and then returned to his shop to allow the line to drain and cool. Upon returning to the film room about 11:00 A.M., the workman discovered a cloud of yellowish smoke in the upper one corner of the room. He emptied a fire extinguisher in the direction of the smoke, but was soon overcome by the fumes and fell to the floor. Revived by a draft of fresh air, he crawled toward the door on hands and knees. A slight explosion flung him through the doorway into a maintenance room, where another workman joined him. Together they made their way through a window and out of the building. Another explosion occurred while the men were still at the window. The custodian of the building spread the alarm.

Alarms were turned in from several locations by telephone. The first was officially recorded at 11:30 A.M., and two others were recorded by 11:44 A.M. Fire companies of East 105th Street just north of Euclid Avenue were the first to respond. When they arrived, most of the building was obscured by a dense cloud of yellowish-brown vapor. Two more alarms brought more fire-fighting equipment and rescue squads. Ladders were raised on each side of the building in an effort to reach and evacuate the people who appeared at the windows. About eight minutes after the arrival of the first fire company, an explosion blew out the skylights and parts of the ceiling of the fourth story. A vast cloud of brown vapor was thus liberated, partially clearing the building of gas. Rescue work then began in earnest. Firemen and volunteers manned stretchers, removed people from the inside, and helped them down the ladders. A rescue squad wearing gas masks tried to enter the front door on the north side, but they were forced out of the building by the concentration of gases. Battalion Chief Michael Graham and members of Hook and Ladder Company 8 entered the building from the roof. Flaming gas was seen through windows in the rear stair shaft and at some of the basement windows. Fire hoses were put into operation in those areas.

Many people died in the north elevator and in the north stairway. Descending the stairway in an effort to escape from the Euclid Avenue entrance, they encountered an ascending mass of frantic people who had found the ground-floor entrance blocked by flames. Many lives were lost in the ensuing melee. Some reached safety by going down ladders from window ledges. Others, by climbing up through the broken skylight, reached the roof of the building and then descended by ladder to the ground.

Dr. A. D. Ruedemann, head of the Department of Ophthalmology, perched on the ledge of his office window on the west side of the fourth floor and supported himself by holding a hot pipe inside the room. He managed to grab a ladder when it reached his level and thus made his way to the ground.[1]

During the confusion of that tragic morning persons trapped within the building were entirely ignorant of the nature of the gas that filled the halls, corridors, and examining rooms. They knew only that it caused severe irritation of the throat and lungs, with coughing and difficult respiration. Those who reached the examining rooms at the sides of the building and closed the doors behind them had a chance of survival. They opened the windows widely and leaned out into the fresh air. When the ladders reached them, many made their way safely to the ground. A few jumped. Dr. Robert S. Dinsmore of the Department of Surgery broke his ankle in a leap from a second floor window on the east side of the building.

A number of Cleveland physicians came to the hospital and spent many hours assisting members of the Clinic staff with their overwhelming task. Living patients were blue and short of breath. It became evident that the problem was one of toxic gas inhalation. Respiration became more difficult, cyanosis increased, and severe pulmonary edema developed. Fluid caused by the irritation of the gas filled the air sacs of the lungs. Many of these persons, including Dr. Locke and Dr. Hunter, died in two or three hours. Some died later that afternoon or that night, among them Mr. William Brown-

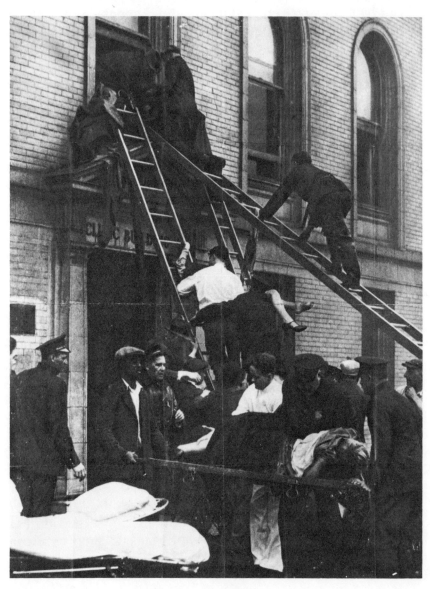

The Disaster, May 15, 1929

low, artist, and Dr. John Phillips, a founder of the Clinic and head of the Medical Department. Phillips reached the ground by a ladder on the east side of the building; he sat for a while on the steps of the church across 93rd Street, and finally was taken by car to his apartment at the Wade Park Manor on East 107th Street. There he became more ill as the afternoon wore on, and about 7:00 P.M. a transfusion team, headed by Dr. Crile, went to his room and performed a transfusion, without avail. Phillips died at about 8:30 P.M. He was only fifty years old at the time, and the loss of such a talented physician and leader was a particularly sad blow to the Clinic and to the medical profession of Cleveland.

On the day after the disaster, Dr. Harvey Cushing, distinguished neurosurgeon in Boston and an old friend of Crile's, came to Cleveland to offer his services. His former assistant, Dr. Charles E. Locke, Jr., who was the first neurologic surgeon on the Clinic staff, 1924–1929, had died of gas inhalation on the previous day. Crile asked his first assistant, Dr. Alexander T. Bunts, to take Cushing around the hospital to see those with any possible neurologic injuries.

Crile and others who had had first-hand experience in treating gassed patients during the war in France commented upon the clinical effects of the gas as being similar to those observed in soldiers who had inhaled phosgene gas ($COCl_2$) at the front. After the disaster, Major General Gilchrist, Chief of the Chemical Warfare Service, came to Cleveland and initiated a thorough investigation of its possible causes. Decomposition of the nitrocellulose film may have been caused (1) by the rise in temperature produced by the leaking and uncovered steam line, (2) by ignition of the film from an incandescent lamp attached to a portable cord close to the shelves, or (3) by a lighted cigarette on or near the films. None of these theories has ever been proved to be the exact cause. The investigations conducted by the Chemical Warfare Service did determine the nature of the gases produced by the burning or decomposition of nitrocellulose films: carbon monoxide and "nitrous fumes" (NO, NO_2, and N_2O_4). Carbon monoxide when breathed in high concentrations causes almost instant death. "Nitrous fumes," comprising most of the brownish gases, became nitric acid on contact with the moisture in the lungs. This led to acute rupture of the alveolar walls, pulmonary congestion, and edema. The Clinic disaster resulted in revision of safety codes adopted worldwide for storing films and led to the use of safety film that would not explode.

After the disaster many problems confronted the two remaining founders. Miss Litta Perkins, executive secretary to the founders and the Board of Trustees and in whose photographic memory existed most of the records of the Foundation, had died. The Clinic building, although still structurally sound, could not be used. The interior was badly damaged, brownish stains were present everywhere, and there was a rumor that lethal fumes were still escaping. There were those who advised razing the building, fearing that patients would never again be willing to enter it. Lower and Crile adopted a wise position. "They'll talk for a while," Crile said, "and then, when they forget it, we'll start again to use the building." That is exactly what happened.

A frame house that stood directly across Euclid Avenue from the Clinic had been used as a dormitory for the girls of Laurel School. This house was made available to the Clinic by Mrs. Lyman, headmistress of the school and a lifelong friend of Crile's. The house was transformed into a temporary clinic. For four days after the disaster the staff and personnel of the Clinic worked unceasingly, aided by carpenters and movers and by a committee of civic leaders headed by Mr. Samuel Mather and Mr. Roger C. Hyatt. Desks, chairs, tables, lamps, x-ray equipment, files, records, and all other necessary material were carried across Euclid Avenue and placed on all three floors of the loaned house. Telephone and power lines were installed. On Monday morning, May 20, 1929, just five days after the disaster, the building was opened for the examination of patients.

Liability insurance coverage for such a loss of life was inadequate, but did provide eight thousand dollars per person plus funeral or hospital expenses. State industrial insurance gave what Crile termed "cold comfort" to the personnel. The medical staff, however, took on the task of paying the families of the members of the staff who died full salary for the first six months and half salary for the second six. The founders, of course, suffered no personal liability, for the Foundation, which owned everything, was a nonprofit corporation and the founders were salaried employees. Expressions of sympathy and offers of financial assistance were received from many Clevelanders and from colleagues or patients as far away as India,

China, and Australia.[2] More than $30,000 poured in as gifts. Then Crile said, "When Lower and I found we still possessed the confidence of the public, of our own staff, and of the members of our institution, we knew we could finance our own way. So, after holding these gifts for a few months of security, we returned them all with their accumulated interest."[3]

After operating in the Laurel School quarters throughout the summer of 1929, the equipment and functions of the Clinic were transferred, in September, to the newly completed addition to the hospital which had just been extended to East 93rd Street. The rooms on several floors were arranged and equipped as examining rooms for out-patients. For the next two years the Clinic's work was carried out here. Although the quarters were cramped, the patients continued to come in increasing numbers.

FOUR

In October 1929, five months after the disaster, the stock market crashed, heralding the great depression of the 1930s. It was at this time, and with three million dollars of lawsuits filed against not only the Foundation but also against Lower and Crile, and the estates of Bunts and Phillips, that the surviving founders decided to build a new three-story Clinic building with foundations to support fourteen stories. It was planned to connect the new building with the one that had been in use since 1921, and to remodel the latter so that it would be difficult for anyone who remembered the disaster and was familiar with the first building to tell which it was. At the time of this decision Crile was 66 years old and Lower was 63. They reasoned that if the court decision went against the Foundation and themselves, all of them would be in bankruptcy and there would be nothing to lose.[1]

The two founders started to raise what money they could to start the new building, but it was not without trepidation that they faced their difficulties. "Every day Ed and I spent the lunch hour in the board room discussing them," Crile wrote. "I was able to convince Ed that we would weather our difficulties; but the next day he would appear so exhausted and excited over a new angle which had occurred to him while he was fighting out the lawsuits overnight, that I told him if someone struck a match near him he would explode. But he was always a joy, appearing one morning with the suggestion that perhaps there would be Christian Scientists on the jury."

From the professional standpoint, 1929 was a good time to start building. The earnings of both Crile and Lower were at their peak.

33

Phillips, lost in the disaster, was replaced as head of the medical division by Dr. Russell L. Haden, a nationally known physician from the University of Kansas who began to create subspecialty departments in internal medicine and who soon developed a large practice in his own specialty, diseases of the blood. There were able young men in all departments, and the reputation and practice of the Clinic were growing rapidly. Indebtedness and the voluntarily assumed burden of paying the salaries of the members of the staff who died in the disaster made it nip and tuck to meet the payroll, and Lower once sent a telegram to Crile, who was attending a meeting in New York, "Just across without reserve."

The financial success of the Clinic at this time depended mainly on the fact that earnings of some of the physicians were more than four times as great as their salaries, the excess going to the Foundation. But in order to borrow the $850,000 required for the new building, Crile and Lower had to put up their personal life insurance policies to guarantee $150,000 of the loan. Three million dollars in lawsuits resulting from the disaster were settled out of court for about $45,000. (The Foundation had no liquid or negotiable assets that would make it worthwhile for the plaintiffs to bring the cases to court.)

In September 1932, in order to help repay the heavy load of debt incurred by the disaster and the cost of the new building, there was a 10 per-cent pay cut for medical staff and for nonprofessional employees. This financial curtailment was accepted graciously, if not enthusiastically, for all were aware of the Clinic's crisis. At that time no one could predict the severity of the great depression that would cloud the years to come. Instead, there was a confident expectation about the future.

"Late in February 1933, while Grace and I were attending a dinner in Cleveland," Crile wrote in his autobiography, "one of the guests, a prominent industrialist and director of one of Cleveland's largest banks, was called to the telephone just as we were seated. He did not return until dinner was nearly over and, when he returned, he seemed deeply perturbed, was without conversation and soon left." The next day the Maryland banks closed; the following day most Cleveland banks announced that only 5 per cent withdrawals were allowed. The economic depression deepened. The banks failed while the Clinic was still heavily in debt. A second 10

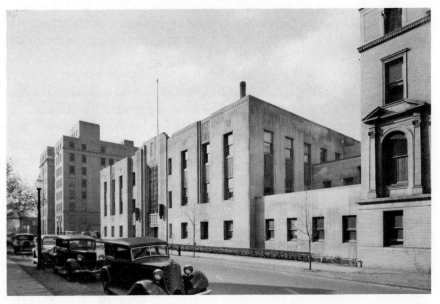

Cleveland Clinic, East 93rd Street   (Left to right) Hospital addition, 1929. Research Building, 1928. Main Clinic (three stories), 1931. Original Clinic Building (S.E. corner showing), 1921   (photographed in 1935)

per cent cut in salaries had been necessary one month before the banks closed. Four months later there was an additional 25 per cent cut. Circulating money had almost ceased to exist, but its absence did not curtail the incidence of disease. The sick still required treatment, and somehow many of them managed to pay something for it. The staff, both professional and nonprofessional, remained loyal, but not always because of their high morale; their choice, in those days of unemployment, lay between a low-paying job and no job at all. The Clinic survived.[2]

In 1934 the depression was still in its depths. Crile's surgical practice still provided the Clinic a major part of its income, and he was now 70 years old. Gradually his interest had shifted from the thyroid surgery that had attracted patients from all over the world to surgery of the adrenal glands, a field that he was exploring in the treatment of such diverse conditions as hypertension, peptic ulcer, epilepsy, hyperthyroidism, and neurocirculatory asthenia. The results of the operations were sometimes promising, but rarely spectacular. The field was so controversial that Crile's personal practice began to shrink. At the same time he underwent operations on his eyes for glaucoma, and soon thereafter, cataracts began to develop.

Fortunately, there were able young associates in the Department of Surgery, including Dr. Robert S. Dinsmore who continued Crile's interest in surgery of the thyroid and breast, and Dr. Thomas E. Jones who had already become nationally famous for abdominal surgery, particularly for cancer of the rectum and colon. The surgical specialties were headed by capable surgeons, and under Haden's leadership the Division of Medicine was expanding rapidly. Therefore, Crile disengaged himself increasingly from conventional surgery and spent more of his time in researches into the energy systems of man and animals, traveling twice to Africa to collect and study the brains, thyroids, and adrenals of various species of African wildlife.[3]

On the way home from Florida in 1941, Dr. and Mrs. Crile and the Clinic's anatomist, Dr. Daniel Quiring, were injured when their airplane hit a tornado and crashed in a swamp near Vero Beach.

"It had been a great day, a manatee was dissected and cast," Dr. Crile wrote, "and we had also stored away in jars the energy organs of a marlin, a sailfish and a barracuda, so we decided to take the early morning plane to Daytona Beach, visit Marineland and catch our train at midnight. This was Quiring's first flight.

"When the steward told us that there were a few thunderheads beyond, Grace remarked that Quiring was going to see a little of every kind of weather. We had left the usual beach route and were flying over marshland that looked like the waterhole country in Africa. The mist became thicker. Suddenly I was conscious of an abrupt vertical upsurge; we had entered the thunderheads and were shrouded in darkness and a violent hail storm, pierced by zigzag lightning that flashed from every bit of metal in the plane. We must have resembled a Christmas tree hurling through space.

"A deafening roar as of a high pressure wind under a powerful drive beat on our ear drums. Blankets, hats, pillows, trays were sucked to the ceiling, then flew in all directions about the cabin. I did not suspect it at the time but we were in an active tornado and were actually observing its mechanism at work. The plane seemed to be whirling. Blackness spun before my eyes. Everything was tipping—I recall how difficult it was to pull my tilting body to the left.

"A lurch! A feeling of gratitude that Grace got off our manuscript to the publisher. Then oblivion!"

Quiring's shoulder was dislocated; Grace Crile suffered two broken ribs, a broken sternum, and a cracked vertebra; and Crile, the most seriously injured of any of the passengers (his seat was at the point where the plane buckled), had three fractures of the pelvis, three broken ribs, and fractures of the transverse processes of two vertebrae as well as severe contusions. Despite these injuries, he was the first to break the silence after the crash. As the chill marsh mire began to rise in the cabin he imagined himself at home in a bathtub. "Grace," he called to his wife, "Grace, would you mind turning on the hot water please?"[4]

Although Crile had remained president of the Foundation until 1940, more and more of the executive duties had been turned over to an administrative board composed of four staff physicians. They were responsible for the professional aspects of administration, and the Board of Trustees, now composed exclusively of laymen, was responsible for properties and finance. Prosperity had returned to the country, and it seemed that the Clinic was out of its financial straits. But there were still other troubles ahead, many of them arising from conflicts of personalities.

In an institution like the Clinic, for many years ruled by the men who had founded it, the transfer of authority to others is always difficult. As soon as the old leaders falter or step down, there ensues a struggle for new leadership. It was at this point that the Board of Trustees, hitherto active largely in support of the founders' decisions, became invaluable. Without the trustees it is doubtful that the institution could have survived. Much of that part of the history of the Clinic is recounted in a later chapter. It is sufficient to say here that able physicians and surgeons are not always the best administrators.

By 1940 Crile's eyesight was failing badly, and he retired from the position of President of the Foundation. His brother-in-law, Mr. Henry S. Sherman, a former industrialist who at the time was president of the Society for Savings (a Cleveland financial institution) and one of the Foundation's trustees, was elected president in his place. Although Lower was still active in an advisory capacity, he, too, was now in his seventies and as anxious as Crile had been to turn over the administrative responsibilities to the next generation.

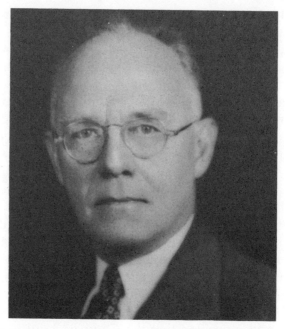

Henry S. Sherman   President, The Cleveland Clinic Foundation, 1942

And so it was that in 1943 Mr. Edward C. Daoust, who had partic-ipated so effectively in the founding of the Clinic, was given the full-time assignment of being President of the Foundation. Sherman became Chairman of the Board of Trustees.[5]

The Foundation had been growing steadily ever since the fi-nancial depression began to lift, and the number of employees had increased from 216 in 1930 to 739 in 1941. In September 1941 the Foundation was able to repay the last $180,000 of its indebtedness. The founders gave up the last of the administrative duties with the comment, "The child has learned to walk." But the road still led uphill.

FIVE

■ TURBULENT SUCCESS
1941–1955

Although it was clear that "the child could walk," the problems of adolescence still had to be met. No firm leadership, either autocratic or democratic, capable of replacing that of the founders had as yet developed. The dominant personalities on the staff were men like Dr. William Mullin, head of the Department of Otolaryngology; Dr. A. D. Ruedemann, head of the Department of Ophthalmology; Dr. Russell L. Haden, head of the Department of Medicine; and Dr. Thomas E. Jones, who replaced Crile as head of the Department of Surgery in 1940. Problems arose as a result of the conflicts among these brilliant and competitive personalities. Sadly, some of their arguments were settled by Dr. Mullin's untimely death in 1935 and by Dr. Ruedemann's resignation from the Clinic in 1947.

One factor that helped to tide over the difficult years of the early 1940s was the sheer weight of work. The military draft had reduced by more than 20 per cent the members of the staff and reduced also the number of residents in training by a third. All this occurred at a time when most of the young physicians of the area were drafted, and thus, many of the patients whom they would normally care for came to the Clinic. Surgical schedules and new-patient registrations rose to an all time high. In 1942 there were 21,500 new patients, and by 1944 the number had increased to 27,900. Everyone was too busy to spend much time discussing administrative affairs. Daoust was an effective chief executive respected by all, and Sherman, chairman of the Board of Trustees, had a unique insight into the problems of the Clinic in which he had been interested since it was founded.

The Clinic's Naval Reserve Unit was called to active duty in the spring of 1942. Two months of training were spent on Pier No. 14 of the Brooklyn Naval Yard, a bleak, barn-like structure in which, as Crile, Jr. recalls, there was very little to do but read *The New York Times*. The Unit then sailed for New Zealand to establish Mobile Hospital No. 4, the first of its kind in the South Pacific.[1] In the Unit were Drs. George Crile, Jr., William J. Engel, A. Carlton Ernstene, W. James Gardner, Roscoe J. Kennedy, Joseph C. Root, William A. Nosik and Edward J. Ryan, as well as Guy H. Williams, Jr. (a neuropsychiatrist from City Hospital, Cleveland) and Don H. Nichols (a Cleveland dentist).

Mobile Hospital No. 4 was based in New Zealand for a year and a half, dealing more with tropical diseases and rehabilitation of the sick than with wounds. Thereafter its officers were dispersed to other stations. As soon as the war was over, those who were in service returned to the Clinic.[2]

Crile was 77 years old when the United States entered World War II. In 1940, after a cataract operation made difficult by a previous operation for glaucoma, he lost an eye. Remaining vision had failed to the point where he could no longer easily recognize people by sight, and he had become subject to occasional spells of unconsciousness. Crile then contracted bacterial endocarditis, and after an illness of several months he died in January 1943.[3]

Crile died with his major quest unfulfilled: he had failed to fathom the unfathomable mystery of life. Nonetheless, he left The Cleveland Clinic Foundation, complete with its own hospital, research, and educational facilities, to stand as a memorial to its founders. The institution's prosperity in the early 1940s made possible many improvements in its facilities. There were troubles ahead, however, and tumultuous times were to characterize the late 1940s.

On January 1, 1943, Daoust retired from his law practice and became the full-time president of The Cleveland Clinic Foundation and its chief administrative officer, responsible to the trustees. He had been associated with the founders and Foundation for more than twenty years. On that date, Sherman became chairman of the Board, and Mr. John Sherwin, whose activities as a trustee were to be so important to the Foundation through the years, joined Daoust and Sherman as the third member of a new executive committee of the Board of Trustees. In Sherwin's words, "While formal meetings were infrequent, luncheon meetings and telephone conversations

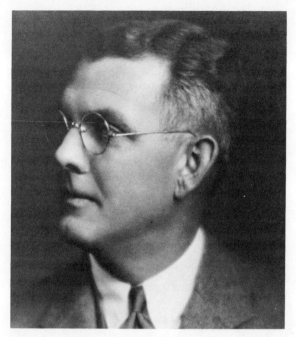

Edward C. Daoust, LL.B.   President, The Cleveland Clinic Foundation, 1943–1947

took place often, and a closer rapport was established with the Administrative Board then composed of Daoust and Drs. Thomas Jones, Russell Haden, A. D. Ruedemann, W. James Gardner, and E. P. McCullagh."

The Administrative Board referred to by Sherwin was established to represent the professional staff. At the same time the new Executive Committee was established. The new Administrative Board had its first meeting in January 1943. The meetings of that body in earlier years have been described as always interesting and frequently almost frightening. Dr. Lower would sometimes leave the meeting trembling visibly. Impressions of the meetings of the Administrative Board were recalled by McCullagh, the youngest member of the Board. "The original Medical Administrative Board was formed in February 1937, and was composed of Dr. Crile, Dr. Lower, Dr. Russell Haden, Dr. Thomas E. Jones, Dr. A. D. Ruedemann, and Dr. Bernard H. Nichols with Mr. Edward Daoust attending. These were exciting meetings, for Dr. Ruedemann, Dr. Jones, and Dr. Haden often reacted suddenly. Sometimes this, added

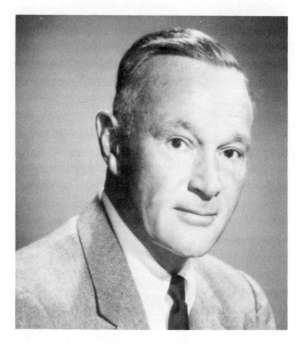

John Sherwin   President, The Cleveland Clinic Foundation, 1948–1957

to a hot temper, would lead close to physical violence. Drs. Haden and Jones, it seemed to me, always disagreed, apparently on general principles. Dr. Ruedemann had no favorites, disagreeing with every-one in turn. This concerned Dr. Crile and Dr. Lower very much, and I'm sure caused them anxiety for fear that no plans for satis-factory Clinic administration were evolving."[4]

The war years and those immediately thereafter brought to the institution both prosperity and professional maturity. Specialization was increasing in both medical and surgical divisions. New-patient registration continued to rise, and in 1947 it was 31,804, nearly three times the number served a decade earlier. This growth necessitated further building, and in 1945 seven stories were added to the new Clinic building. One year later a wing was added to the hospital, connecting the hospital to the research building.[5] These post-war years needed the steady hand of Daoust in the administration of a growing organization, and his accidental death in June 1947 was a serious blow to the Foundation. The airliner on which Daoust was a passenger crashed into a mountain top. All on board were killed.

The administrative crisis precipitated by the death of Daoust was met promptly by the trustees. Sherwin's own account states that on the morning following the airplane crash, Lower, Sherman, and Sherwin met to determine how best Daoust's responsibilities could be assumed. There had already been many discussions among trustees about how to administer the Foundation after the retirement of its founders. Conversations had taken place with the management consulting firm of Booz, Allen and Hamilton with an idea to engage that firm in a study of the Clinic and its operations and to obtain recommendations from them.

Sherman, Sherwin and Lower agreed to recommend to the Board of Trustees that

- the position of president should be left vacant for the time being
- the responsibilities of the president be assumed by the Executive Committee
- Sherwin become chairman of the Executive Committee
- Messrs. John R. Chandler, Benjamin F. Fiery, Walter M. Halle, and John C. Virden, all of whom had just recently been elected trustees, join Sherman and Sherwin on the Executive Committee
- the Executive Committee in conjunction with the Administrative Board employ Booz, Allen and Hamilton to make a study and recommend
  a) how the Foundation should be administered and
  b) how the compensation of the professional staff should be determined.

These recommendations were adopted by the Board of Trustees on June 26, 1947, and a new Administrative Board membership composed of Drs. Dickson, Ernstene, Gardner, Jones, and Netherton was appointed. That same day the staff assembled specifically to learn of these actions.

During the ensuing four months the Executive Committee and Administrative Board met almost weekly, usually from five o'clock in the afternoon through dinner and then on to ten o'clock or after. Representatives of Booz, Allen and Hamilton attended most of these meetings. These men reviewed the entire operation of the institution

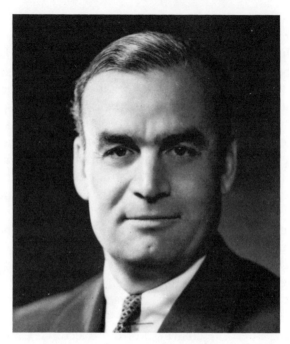

Clarence M. Taylor   Executive Director, 1948–1955

and developed a plan for the organization and operation of the Foundation. The plan of August 14, 1947, had the unanimous support of the trustees and the Administrative Board. It was during the last year of Lower's life that Booz, Allen and Hamilton gathered data for their report to the trustees. The idea of spending money for this sort of thing came to annoy him, and Lower, the ever frugal and conservative founder, finally refused to talk with the management consultants.[6]

It was during these sessions that everyone realized the need for an administrative head. A search started for such a person, and in October Mr. Clarence M. Taylor, recently retired as executive vice president of Lincoln Electric Company, was invited to become executive director. He assumed the office on January 1, 1948, but spent the balance of 1947 acquainting himself with the Booz, Allen and Hamilton report and the operation of the Clinic. Sherwin continued to assume the duties and responsibilities of executive director until Taylor's arrival.

The plan of organization and operation and the appointment

of Taylor were announced at a special meeting of the staff.[7] Jones described the plan as the staff's "Magna Charta" and the new executive director as a "welder—formerly of metals, now of people." Both statements proved to be accurate. Although some staff members had misgivings, the plan was, on the whole, enthusiastically accepted. That administration and policy were the responsibility of lay trustees and that the entire professional operation was the responsibility of a professional staff organization were principles formally brought into being by the plan. It was at this time that Sherwin was elected president of the Foundation.

A member of the professional staff observed many years later that one of the most extraordinary events in the history of the Clinic took place in this period.[8] Without salary or remuneration of any kind, the Executive Committee of the Board of Trustees, and Sherwin in particular, devoted many hours a week to meeting with representatives of the professional staff and with the management consultants. The issue was how to manage the Clinic. All of the men on the board were busy executives with full-time careers of their own. At this critical time they were not figure-head trustees. They shouldered the full responsibility of their office, bringing to it the organizational skills, the patience, and the understanding that characterize top-flight executives. To these men the Clinic owes an enormous debt of gratitude.[9]

At the time of Daoust's death in 1947, there was little harmony among the members of the staff and no organization in which democratic processes could function. The president had been empowered to conduct the Foundation's business affairs; each department head was an autocrat in charge of the professional policies of his own department, and the sometimes tumultuous sessions of the Administrative Board have already been described. The composition of the board was altered in 1947 with Ruedemann's resignation from the staff, and in 1949 with the retirement of Haden and the death of Jones. Jones fell dead in the surgeons' locker room of a ruptured aneurysm of the heart. Under changing leadership, the climate was improving for the development of a more democratic organization of the professional staff.

Sometimes aging renders leadership too rigid in outlook. Several persons remaining in key positions were in their sixties. In the early 1950s there was hardening of the lines of authority. One department chairman said that you couldn't run a department and win a popularity contest, too. Some of the younger members of the staff began to feel that there was no democratic process allowing them to register either protests or preferences. In those days, one of the ethical principles of the American Medical Association stated that "A physician should not dispose of his professional attainments or services to a hospital, body, or organization, group or individual, by whatever name called or however organized under terms or conditions which permit exploitation of the physician for financial profit of the agency concerned." This historic principle made it unethical for any physician to permit a third party to intervene in the relationship between the doctor and his patient. Members of the staff were also members of the A.M.A., and some began to feel insecure under a plan of organization that seemed sometimes to infringe upon this ethical principle.[10]

With the purpose of investigating this and related problems, the trustees of the Foundation and the Professional Policy Committee of the Clinic met on October 13, 1954, and appointed a Medical Survey Committee.[11] After several months of careful deliberation and consultation with every member of the staff, the Medical Survey Committee issued a report recommending changes in both administrative and professional affairs of the Foundation.[12]

The Medical Survey Committee suggested that many of the Clinic's problems could be solved if the trustees delegated certain responsibilities to an elected board of governors composed of members of the professional staff.[13] They recommended that a planning committee of trustees and staff be charged to study the administrative structure of the Clinic. The Board of Trustees accepted the recommendation.[14]

The Planning Committee met frequently during the summer of 1955, and as a result of its deliberations a new plan of organization was adopted by the Board of Trustees. The new organization provided that all professional matters pertaining to the practice of medicine be under the jurisdiction of a board of governors. Provision was made also to form elected committees within the divisions of medicine, surgery, and pathology.[15] These divisional committees were to act under the authority of a board of governors in the management of professional affairs within their domain.[16] The proposed plan delegated responsibility for medical practice to a board of governors to be composed of seven members of the professional staff.[17] These were to be elected by the staff for staggered terms of five years. To prevent self-perpetuation, no member would be eligible for reelection for one year after expiration of the term. To prevent election of members of the board by cliques, an indirect method would be employed. Each year a nominating committee would be elected by the staff. After deliberation this committee would nominate a member of the staff to fill each vacancy. The entire staff then would vote on the nominees, and if 60 per cent approved each candidate, he or she would be elected.[18] Only twice in the years since this system was introduced has the staff failed to support the nominating committee's candidates.

Since the Division of Research was supported by endowment funds, earnings of the Clinic, and outside grants, its administrative problems were to be the responsibility of the Board of Trustees. For this purpose the Committee on Research Policy and Administration was established. A separate committee, the Research Projects Committee, appointed by the Board of Governors from the members of the Division of Research and from members of the clinical divisions who had special knowledge or interest in research problems, was put in control of all research projects undertaken by members of the clinical divisions. The long-range program of research, devoted largely to the study of hypertension and arteriosclerosis, remained under the control of the Director of Research, Dr. Irvine H. Page, who reported only to the Board of Trustees.[19]

As a memorial to Bunts, an educational foundation was established and named for him some years after his death. The same Board of Trustees that directed The Cleveland Clinic Foundation also directed the Educational Foundation. The original endowments and also the profits of the Cleveland Clinic Pharmacy (incorporated as a taxable, profit-making company) supported the Educational Foundation.

The report of the Planning Committee was a document of enormous significance with far-reaching consequences. Many issues were addressed. The months of effort in 1955 were rewarded by a truly new system of governance for the Foundation. At a meeting of the professional staff it was unanimously recommended that the professional members of the Planning Committee nominate the first Board of Governors.[20]

SIX

■ TRUSTEES AND GOVERNORS 1955–1984

Issues of Management, Growth, and Control

The Board of Governors was established in 1955 and in the years to follow assumed increasing responsibility for the direction of the Foundation. There have been three chairmen of the Board of Governors during these twenty-nine years, each of whom made lasting contributions to the institution. Dr. Fay A. LeFevre served from the beginning of the era of the Board of Governors through 1968, and then Dr. Carl E. Wasmuth succeeded him as chairman, serving through most of 1976. The third and present chairman is Dr. William S. Kiser. The challenges, issues, and opportunities of each administration characterize these periods of leadership as do the personalities of the leaders themselves.

If after the establishment of the Board of Governors there is an evolving theme, it is the role of increasing managerial responsibility assumed by the Board of Governors. The trustees have necessarily maintained public accountability, but they have given to the Board of Governors many responsibilities. The ultimate responsibilities of defining institutional purpose, acquiring and selling property, the compensation of the staff, and budgetary approval still rest with the trustees.

After twenty-nine years of operation, one can look back with some amazement at the success of the plan of organization as developed by the Planning Committee in 1955. During the early years of this period only minor changes were made. The original plan stated that the chairman must be a voting member of the Board of

49

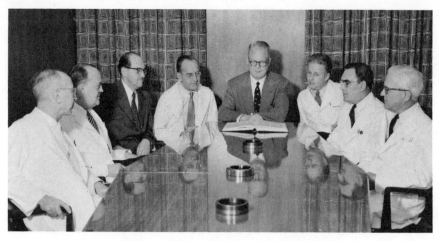

Board of Governors, 1956. Left to right: Drs. W. James Gardner, E. Perry Mc-Cullagh, Walter J. Zeiter (Executive Secretary), Irvine H. Page, Fay A. LeFevre (Chairman), George Crile, Jr., A. Carlton Ernstene, William J. Engel

Governors. With the recommendation of the staff, this was amended so that any member of the staff could be elected chairman. The Board of Governors from its inception was able to mold a group of individuals, highly trained in their specialties, so that they could work together unselfishly. This achievement is attributable largely to a democratic system of selecting governors.

THE LEFEVRE YEARS, 1955–1968

Little did the gentlemen who first met as governors in December 1955 realize the magnitude of the responsibilities they would come to assume and the importance of the decisions they and future Boards of Governors were to make. And little did LeFevre realize that he would serve as chairman for the next thirteen exciting and formative years. Following months of discussion and deliberation, the Planning Committee had recommended, and the Board of Trustees had approved, that responsibility for all professional matters be delegated to the Board of Governors. How this change came about and what prompted it has been related in the previous chapter.

It became the responsibility of the board to plan and coordinate all professional activities. Among its important duties were to ap-

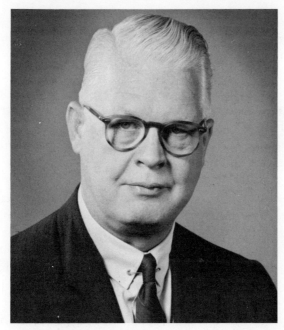

Fay A. LeFevre, M.D.   Chairman, Board of Governors, 1955–1968

point, promote, or release members of the professional staff. With the growth of the institution this became an increasingly important and difficult matter. It was also necessary for members of the board to review criticisms and complaints concerning relationships with patients, and to initiate corrective measures. In addition it was the board's responsibility to review and establish fees for professional services and to review at regular intervals the financial results of professional activities. As the Clinic expanded, planning and policy-making were tasks that took increasing amounts of time. The success of these efforts required the cooperation of trustees and governors, working together.

LeFevre had for many years served as a director of the Chesapeake and Ohio Railroad and was knowledgeable in business and finance. As chairman of the Board of Governors it was his wish to continue a part-time practice of medicine. He believed that by keeping in touch with professional problems he would be in a better position to understand them. For some time it was possible for LeFevre to do this, and he found it both satisfying and stimulating.

"It was also a great protective mechanism for me," he said. "When things got 'too hot' in the first floor administrative offices, Janet Getz would call me and say that my patients were ready on the third floor. This gave me an ideal opportunity to excuse myself. Likewise, when some patients became too longwinded, I could politely say that an urgent problem had occurred in the administrative office that would require my immediate attention. This best of two worlds did not last long, however, for it was necessary to spend more and more time in the administrative office."

In the '50s and '60s there were those, particularly among the trustees, who thought that the administration of medical affairs by the Board of Governors would not succeed. The responsibility for professional affairs had been delegated to a professional group, and business affairs were under the direction of a business manager. The weakness in this arrangement was that no one person had the final authority to make a major decision when professional and business issues were joined.

Throughout this era the trustees kept a tight rein on the management of the Clinic by the placement of their representatives in key authoritative roles—those of business manager and hospital administrator. Nonetheless, the Board of Governors had plenty to do. There were pressures to provide new facilities, to expand existing services, and to subspecialize clinical practice to meet both the demands of patients and the opportunities of practice. These pressures led to the growth of the professional staff and ultimately to the need to acquire property and build new facilities. The impetus for these changes (growth and increasing numbers of patients) lay with the professional staff, but it was for the Board of Governors to interpret and organize the needs of patients and staff so that the trustees could understand and respond.

The trustees were ably led between 1956 and 1968 first by John Sherwin and then by George Karch. James A. Hughes became chairman in 1969 and, except for the period when Arthur S. Holden, Jr. served in that post (1973 and 1974), has continued his leadership to the present day. The first members of the professional staff to serve on the Board of Trustees were Drs. W. James Gardner, Fay A. LeFevre, and Irvine H. Page, and since 1956 there have always been members of the staff included on that body. This representation quickened the tempo of decision making and such planning as was done in those days, but this is not to say that decision making was easy. The investment in new property, buildings, and equipment led to an increased volume of work and therefore to increases in revenues, staff, and the total number of employees. It was to the trustees that the Board of Governors looked for authorization of its plans and allocation of the money necessary to fund them. The money for all these projects of expansion was in hand, that is to say there was no debt financing, and funds set aside from operational revenues were adequate for payment in full. Long-term financial obligations were to be useful instruments only in a later era.

Several construction projects were undertaken in the LeFevre era that were to lay to rest a nagging issue for both doctors and trustees. The issue was whether or not to abandon the inner city location of the Clinic and move the entire operation into or even beyond the eastern suburbs of Cleveland. A bequest of Martha Holden Jennings built the Education Building, and that was followed by additions to the Clinic and Hospital buildings and by the construction of a hotel (now called the West Clinic) to lodge patients and their families from out of town. Parking garages were built, and the trustees authorized the acquisition of real estate adjoining the Clinic to allow for future expansion. The Clinic was to remain in the city.

The Board of Governors made a decision in December 1965 that was to have an impact far beyond what might then have been imagined. This was the decision to close the obstetrical service. Behind this move was mounting pressure for space and facilities to carry forward the work in cardiology and cardiac surgery. Something had to give, and in the competition for institutional support the winner was the program in heart disease. A declining national birth rate made the decision easier.

The nature of obstetrical services in American hospitals, as decreed by the Joint Commission on Accreditation of Hospitals, was to isolate them from much of the hospital. Delivery rooms, newborn nurseries, and the rooms for mothers were separated from the surgical patients and the general operating rooms in the Cleveland Clinic. Into this area, Drs. Effler and Groves moved the Department of Thoracic and Cardiovascular Surgery, and thus were consolidated the operating rooms, recovery room, intensive care unit, and convalescent wards of what was to become the most productive and the most renowned department in the Division of Surgery.

In the LeFevre era, there were two sets of issues destined to generate conflict in matters of governance and authority. The conflict was inevitable because Mr. Richard A. Gottron, the business manager of the Clinic, and Mr. James G. Harding, the administrator of the Hospital, reported to the Board of Trustees and not to the Board of Governors or its chairman. Sitting ex officio with the Board of Governors was helpful to Gottron and Harding in the exercise of their duties and provided them the opportunity to be sympathetic with the wishes and the ideas of the governors, but their sympathy could never be expected to endure.

The first set of issues had to do with institutional growth and its capital cost. The trustees were anxious lest the ambitions of the staff set the institution on a breakneck pace of development in which the prudence of businesslike standards could easily be cast aside. Gottron nourished that fear, and his pessimism respecting the growth of the Foundation irreconcilably alienated him from the governors by the summer of 1968.[1]

The second and more subtle sets of issues had to do with management, authority, and control in what by then had become a large enterprise. By 1968 it had been nearly thirteen years since the first meeting of the Board of Governors, and that body had successfully faced matters of policy, planning, and professional practice. With LeFevre's leadership, the governors had worked together and had discovered themselves to represent the strength of the professional staff. Governance of the organization was beginning to take on a new meaning. The governors could not take the next step, however, without the willingness of the trustees to recognize them as a responsible body, delegating to them through their chairman the operations of the Clinic and the Hospital. The dialogue between trustees and governors in the summer of 1968 led to that next step. Mr. James H. Nichols replaced Gottron as business manager, and both he and Harding were to report to the chairman of the Board of Governors.[2] LeFevre, who was ready to retire, would be succeeded by a chairman who was destined to function like a chief executive officer of a large corporation.

THE WASMUTH YEARS, 1969–1976

The modern era began with Wasmuth's tenure as chairman of the Board of Governors. The physician manager emerged at that time, and the tasks addressed by this new breed of doctor are similar to those faced today by executives in industry, government, or education. Wasmuth was head of the Department of Anesthesiology and president of the American Society of Anesthesiologists when he was appointed chairman of the Board of Governors. He had been a general practitioner of medicine, and after board certification in anesthesiology Wasmuth had acquired a law degree.

In his first year as chairman, Wasmuth faced an enormous amount of work to be done and no one to whom he would delegate authority.[3] Early in his administration both Nichols and Harding resigned. The governors were all busy practitioners and the trustees no longer had a resident manager, so Wasmuth assumed personal authority in a way that had not existed since the early days when day-to-day direction was provided by the founders themselves. It was essential that he devote full time to the office of the chairman, and therefore Wasmuth gave up clinical practice and his post as head of the Department of Anesthesiology.

During the LeFevre years, the west wing of the Hospital was added, but scarcely had it opened when the build-up of patient demand made clear the need for more beds in the very near future. Plans were therefore developed for the South Hospital addition and a new Research Building. Moreover, the need arose to build a hotel and two parking garages. How to finance the development was an important question in the early Wasmuth years.

Cash on the barrelhead had been a traditional way of paying for things, but there would no longer be enough money for that way of doing business. The investments required were simply too big, and the operating needs of a large organization required enormous amounts of available cash. The proposal Wasmuth presented to the trustees was that long-term borrowing from local banks pay the construction costs beyond those that could be met by cash outlays from current operating funds. And so it was that debt financing, in principle, was agreed upon by governors and trustees.

To minimize debt, heavy commitments of operating funds were made to these new projects in the early 1970s, and this created some difficult times. Money was in short supply for many routine needs, because an insufficient amount was borrowed and the term of the loan was too short. During this time the government imposed a period of price and wage controls, and there was once again a feeling

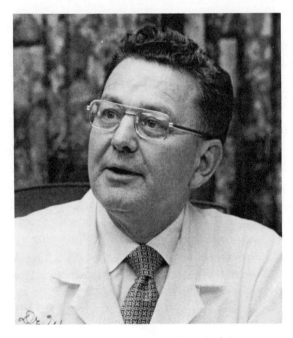

Carl E. Wasmuth, M.D., J.D.   Chairman, Board of Governors, 1969–1976

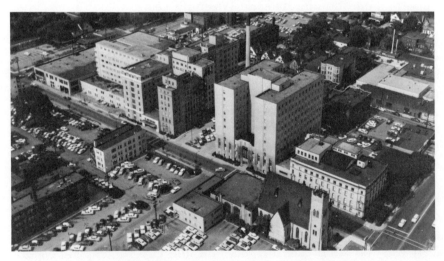

Aerial view of The Cleveland Clinic Foundation, 1969

among the staff that they were being exploited. The memories of these years shaped the opinion of the doctors for a long time to come, and their feelings were not easily assuaged. Yet, throughout the 1970s the Clinic thrived, in large measure because of the expansion that allowed more and more work to be done. It is perhaps to be regretted that the financing of those projects was as stressful as it was. However, important lessons were learned that aided governors and trustees to finance the expansion of the 1980s. But more of that in due course. It is very much to the credit of Wasmuth that he courageously and confidently launched the expansion of the 1970s, that he envisioned the Clinic as the national health resource that it became, and that he set about to persuade governors and trustees that all available neighborhood real estate should be acquired.

As the Clinic leveled squalor on the property it bought, or razed familiar buildings to replace them with new ones, the Clinic was becoming conspicuous. People talked about it increasingly, and not only about how the neighborhood might be improved but also about how big the Clinic was getting. In brief, the Clinic was forced to deal with its image, and this was done with difficulty. The days were over when an organization could be aloof from public sentiment and pay no attention to how and why the public's perceptions, and therefore feelings, were established. During the Wasmuth years the trustees experienced more exposure to adverse public feeling than at any other time before or since in the history of the Clinic.

There were two public arenas into which the Clinic was thrust in the late 1960s and well into the 1970s: social responsibility and city politics. Trustees and governors had little or no experience shaping opinions held by such diverse publics as the neighborhood, minority groups, the professional community, health care planning agencies, Blue Cross, Blue Shield, and the Cleveland City Council. And yet the resolution of issues such as the availability of medical care for the indigent,[4] zoning changes and neighborhood use variances, the building of a viaduct over a city street, the closing of East 93rd Street, and the number of additional hospital beds[5] all depended upon the attitudes and opinions held by these constituencies. To complicate matters further, issues in the public arena were naively approached without policies and techniques for public information and education. Virtually anything at the interface of the

Clinic and the public was dealt with *ad hoc* and in ways that could not help but be perceived as manipulative. In 1976 this perception was addressed through private inquiry by a blue ribbon committee of governors and trustees under the chairmanship of Hughes, and finally certain improprieties were addressed by the judicial system. The harmony with which the trustees and governors worked together in this difficult time was a model of responsible behavior on the part of each and a tribute to the integrity of the Foundation.

After 1968 the scope of responsibility given to the chairman of the Board of Governors was burdensome. The Board of Governors was now in charge not only of all professional matters in the Clinic, the Hospital, the Research Division, and the Educational Foundation, but of operational matters in these areas as well.[6] The chairman, therefore, could scarcely be expected to be conversant with the myriad of details essential to the progress and the interaction of all these entities, even with the most valiant effort. Moreover, the Board of Trustees needed increasing amounts of his time and attention and so did a vast array of public interests. Wasmuth carried this burden with energy and enthusiasm for almost eight years before retiring, but he, the trustees, and the governors realized the need for another person to understudy him. So much was now resting on the chairman that a backup in administration was needed—some trusted and well-liked member of the staff. A search committee identified Dr. William S. Kiser, a governor and urologic surgeon, as a person with administrative talents and a willingness to become a physician manager. This was to prove a very fortunate choice for the future of the Clinic. Kiser became Wasmuth's assistant and, like Wasmuth, he knew that the demands of administration would allow no time for clinical practice. To see a valued colleague and friend give up clinical practice to develop a career as a manager was difficult for many of the professional staff to accept. However, the professional staff had come a long way in the struggle to have a strong voice in the direction of the institution; the Board of Governors was established to provide the governance that represented the doctors; and perhaps it was only natural that one of them should specialize in business affairs just as others were led into areas of scientific or clinical specialization. The latter kind of commitment was, after all, something that might easily be comprehended by the staff. Kiser enrolled in the Advanced Management Program at Harvard, where he was the second physician to complete that distinguished course of study, and in due course he was named vice chairman of the Board of Governors and placed in charge of operations.

By 1974 when the new south wing of the Hospital was to open and wherein the main Hospital lobby would be located as well as the offices of the Board of Governors, there had developed a restlessness of the professional staff. They felt the Board of Governors to be estranged from a growing number of the staff's concerns. This seeming alienation was symbolized by the removal of Wasmuth's office and the board room from the first floor of the Main Clinic Building. Nearly all the staff had walked by that door many times a day for several years, and the new, remote, and well furnished location served to represent an aloofness.

The staff was larger by far than it had been in the 1950s and early 1960s, and the issues that faced the governing boards did indeed eclipse some of the professional and personal matters that the staff felt should be addressed by the governors. The governors met only once a week, and Wasmuth did not have time for these concerns, so the Board of Governors appointed Dr. Leonard L. Lovshin, chairman of the Department of Internal Medicine and a former governor, to function as mediator and liaison person to the professional staff. He was given the title of Director of Professional Affairs. Lovshin's amiability, popularity, and seniority were an asset, but the job was not designed to allow the director to influence policy-making and decisions at the highest level. Recognizing this, some time thereafter the governors took another step to augment the administrative staff that Wasmuth sorely needed. They appointed one of their own number to be vice chairman for Professional Affairs.

The man selected was Dr. Shattuck W. Hartwell, Jr., a plastic surgeon, a member of the Board of Governors, and a member of the Board of Trustees. Hartwell and Lovshin worked together through the end of the Wasmuth years and into the Kiser era when Lovshin retired. By that time the Office of Professional Affairs had evolved into a full-time functioning extension of the Board of Governors assisting the professional divisions in matters of staffing, recruitment, benefits, policy, and mediation. In time, the title of Vice Chairman of the Board of Governors would be reserved for the chief operating officer, and the title of Vice Chairman for Professional Affairs would become Director, Professional Staff Affairs. Nonetheless, the physician manager emerges as a specialist and an essential player in the governance of the Clinic during the Wasmuth years. We shall see how in the Kiser era the position of physician manager becomes even more important.

Wasmuth and his board recognized the need for specialists in management. The legal and financial offices were ably staffed, but personnel matters were not administered in ways that were up-to-date for an organization that by then numbered 3,500 employees. The institution had grown too rapidly for existing systems to keep pace, and the modern practice of personnel management required an experienced expert. Mr. Douglas A. Saarel was such a person, and for three years (1974–1977) he was director of Human Resources. Saarel had a great influence on personnel practices at the Clinic. His systems and organization are still in place.

THE KISER YEARS, 1976–

When Kiser succeeded Wasmuth as chairman of the Board of Governors, the Board of Governors had been in existence for 20 years. Governance of the Clinic was evolving over that period of time, and the power and obligations of the governors in 1976 were distinctly more than they were in 1956. The modern period began with Wasmuth. With Kiser's leadership the governors systematized management to an extent that went far beyond what was begun in the 1968–1976 period.

The utilization of committees had long been a practice at the Clinic. Committees involved large numbers of the staff in all the various assignments that committees undertake. Although there would be occasions when a decision by the governors might appear arbitrary, the input of committees was respected. A continuing refinement of committee function and responsibility has been characteristic of the post-1976 period.

By 1982, the day-to-day operation of the institution required the cooperative function of the division chairmen whose role as managers had become well defined. This cooperation was formalized by the creation of a committee of the division chairmen called the Management Group. The Management Group reports to the Board of Governors through its chairman, Dr. John J. Eversman. Eversman, an endocrinologist, is the chief operating officer of the

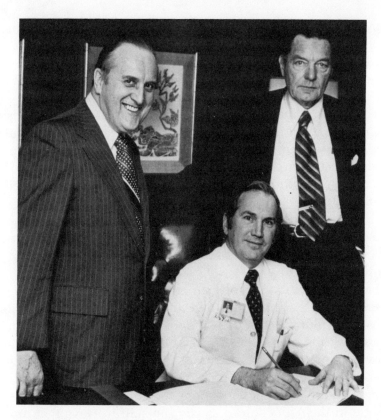

(Left to right)   Harry T. Marks, President, The Cleveland Clinic Foundation, 1975–1980. William S. Kiser, M.D., Chairman, Board of Governors from 1976. James A. Hughes, Chairman, Board of Trustees, 1969–1972 and from 1975.

Clinic and the vice chairman of the Board of Governors. Kiser, Eversman, and Hartwell are members of the Board of Trustees and its Executive Committee ex officio.

Differences between Wasmuth and Kiser may be traced, in part, to the way each perceived himself as a chief executive: Wasmuth chose to function as a chief executive officer with central control; Kiser encouraged decentralization of operating responsibility among a group of physician managers (the division chairmen) and lay administrators. These managers are still accountable, via the chief operating officer, to the Board of Governors and its chairman (the policy makers).[7] It is, in turn, the chairman of the Board of Governors whom the Board of Trustees holds responsible for the operational management of the Foundation. The openness between the two bodies and the representation of the doctors on the Board of Trustees have created a working atmosphere that may well be envied by other institutions and is a credit to the Kiser administration.

The distribution of operational responsibility to the divisions and the departments meant that preparation of the annual budget would be dependent upon input from the chairmen of divisions and departments. At first this was difficult, for lack of experience, but by 1979 budget-setting was becoming an orderly process for all the chairmen. This kind of participation is typical of the involvement that the Board of Governors now expects from the staff, in the belief that a strong professional staff is critical to the continued success of the Foundation and that a strong professional staff must be given responsibility.

Large organizations tend naturally to be hierarchical. The titles of department chairman and division chairman indicate responsibilities and influence, but they are not autocratic; this would not be tolerated by the staff. The Board of Governors is the highest authority on issues that do not require action of the Board of Trustees, and access to the board is a right of every member of the staff. The staff created the Board of Governors; the governors must, therefore, continue in their function to satisfy the staff in ways that are also responsible to the Foundation.

Beginning in 1975 the relationship of the staff to the Board of Governors was formalized in a process known as the Annual Professional Review. This relationship is linked to an annual appraisal of the professional departments and of each of the members within the departments.[8] The reviews, organized by the Office of Professional Staff Affairs, are conducted throughout the year and provide the doctors an opportunity to discuss their attainments, plans, career goals, or departmental issues with representatives of the Board of Governors. More than anything else the custom of the Annual Professional Review keeps the division chairmen and the Board of Governors in touch with the staff, blunts the tendency to hierarchy, and is a potent check on the performance of departmental leadership. The Compensation Committee of the Board of Trustees is apprised of the annual reviews. The reviews have become a well established part of professional life in the Clinic.

There is no better example of cooperation between the Board of Trustees and the Board of Governors than the long-range planning that was begun in 1979. The demand for services, increasing technology, and growth of the staff led to crowded facilities. At that time there was launched a well organized effort to assess where the Clinic would be through the 1980s and 1990s, and this effort drew upon the cooperation of virtually the entire staff. A Minneapolis consulting firm, Hamilton and Associates, worked with the staff and governing bodies to develop a report. The volume of clinical practice, the impact of health care technology, marketing and demographics, beds, facilities, and growth of the staff were among many difficult issues that took two entire years to work through.[9]

Concurrent with the planning effort were studies to determine the best way to finance the growth of the Clinic. Forecasting the need for money involved much careful work, ably done by Robert J. Fischer, treasurer of the Foundation, and Gerald E. Wolf, controller of the Foundation. Their predictions were that an enormous amount of money would be needed over a ten-year period for a new clinical building, another addition to the hospital, a connecting overhead viaduct, parking facilities, equipment, and site development of a much expanded clinic. The experience of the early 1970s (when so much revenue was committed to capital investment) suggested that long-term bonds would be the best way to finance these projects. The Board of Trustees authorized the sale of $228,000,000 in bonds, and in June 1982, all the bonds were quickly sold. It was the largest private financing project in the history of American health care and a tribute to the national esteem enjoyed by the Cleveland Clinic and to the skills of its planners and the financial officers. One year later, refinancing of this debt was successful at the more favorable interest rates then prevailing.

Notable in the Kiser years has been the establishment of offices of public affairs, development, archives, staff benefits, and health systems planning. Wasmuth was farsighted to see the need for a full-time architect, planner, and an internal auditor, and he made appointments to fill these positions. Kiser advanced the idea that a support staff of administrative specialists was essential to the continuing development of the Clinic, and the contributions that these offices have made are proof that he was correct.

Since the days of the founders, nursing services in the Clinic had been in traditional relationships with the doctors. In the '60s and particularly in the '70s, nursing practice in the United States

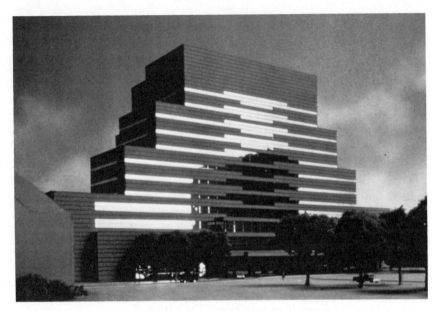

Architect's rendering of new Clinic, 1985

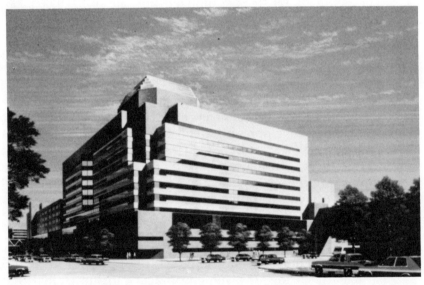

Architect's rendering of new Hospital, 1985

was much affected by two developments: the feminist movement and the increasing subspecialization of clinical practice (to include the rapid deployment of technology in medicine generally and in particular the development of critical care medicine in hospitals). The old relationships with physicians were changing, and nurses were in short supply. Staffing the Cleveland Clinic with adequate numbers of nurses was difficult in this period, as it was for nearly all hospitals. Mr. James E. Lees, Director of Operations, gave much thought to the role of the professional nurse in the future of the Clinic, and a decision was made to bring into the highest managerial council the leadership of nursing. Since the reorganization of 1968 and the beginning of the Wasmuth era there had been no nursing hierarchy in the traditional sense. Kiser realized the importance of nursing with a voice equal to the division chairmen in the key operating committee, the Management Group. The search for a person to provide this kind of leadership resulted in the appointment in 1981 of Sharon L. Danielsen, R.N., as administrative director of nursing services.

In this chronicle of the years 1956–1984, there remain two other administrative innovations at the Clinic since 1976 that are of special significance: the Office of Fund Development and the Office of Public Affairs. Both were adaptations to the changing environment: a decrease in the amount of money available for education and research and a burgeoning public awareness of the Clinic.[10]

The mission of The Cleveland Clinic Foundation, restated and clarified during the Kiser years, is to care for patients "in a setting of research and education." To provide this setting would be increasingly expensive, and the research of Fischer and Wolf had made it clear that in the future the funds from operational revenues and endowment would not be adequate to the task. Additional funds for education and research would have to be obtained from gifts, bequests, and foundation support, and so the Board of Trustees authorized an Office of Fund Development.

Earlier in this history we saw how ill-prepared the Clinic was to manage public perceptions of the Clinic. Trustees and governors agreed that attention to public affairs was important not only for the Clinic but for the public. Large amounts of information that would be of interest and value to the public lay within the institution. How to manage this information required the skill of an expert. A task force studied internal and external communications, and its report led to a search for such an expert. In 1980, Mr. Frank J. Weaver became the Clinic's first director of what now is the Division of Public Affairs.

The Cleveland Clinic Foundation is now sixty-three years old. At no time in its past has it been stronger. The trustees and governors understand more clearly than ever their responsibilities in fulfilling the mission of the institution.[11] Of the 7,200 employees of the Foundation, nearly 400 are members of the professional staff. But the staff is more than a group of employees; the system of governance that has developed over the past sixty-three years involves the participation of the staff, providing them the opportunities for leadership and influence that will assist the Board of Trustees to shape the future of the organization. This system is the best example to date of how trustees and governors can truly act as a unit.

SEVEN

■ ". . . BETTER CARE OF THE
SICK . . ."

Division of Medicine

Dr. John Phillips, the only internist among the four founders, became chief of the Division of Medicine. The eight years between 1921 and his untimely death in the disaster was a period of transition in the way medicine was practiced. The trend from house calls to an office practice had begun. By inclination and experience Phillips was a family physician. Even after he was head of the Division of Medicine he continued to make house calls and to treat patients with diverse disorders.[1] As a founder, he recognized the value of specialization not only between surgery and medicine, but within medicine itself. Thus in 1921, Dr. Henry John was assigned the field of diabetes and supervision of the clinical laboratories; in 1923 Dr. Earl W. Netherton became head of the Department of Dermatology; and in 1929 Dr. E. Perry McCullagh started the Department of Endocrinology. The rest of the medical staff practiced general medicine.[2]

In September 1930, a year and a half after the death of Phillips, Dr. Russell L. Haden, Professor of Experimental Medicine at the University of Kansas School of Medicine, was appointed chief of the Division of Medicine. There was a significant difference between those two able physicians. Phillips had been interested primarily in the clinical aspects of disease, and in his eight years at the Clinic 26 of his papers were published, 23 of which were concerned primarily with unusual cases or the diagnosis or treatment of various diseases. Haden had 26 papers published within five years after coming to the Clinic. Only three concerned case reports or treatment; the other

67

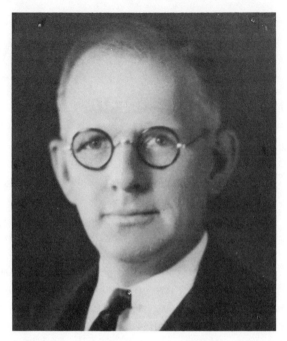

Russell L. Haden, M.D.   Chief of Medicine, 1930–1949

23 were descriptions of laboratory innovations or attempts to define the causes or interrelations of various diseases. In short, Haden was the Clinic's first representative of the modern, laboratory-oriented medical scientist.

Haden's interests spanned the entire field of internal medicine, but he was primarily a hematologist. He made many important contributions to the knowledge of diseases of the blood and blood-forming organs, the most historic being the discovery of the sphero-cytic shape of red blood cells in what was then called congenital hemolytic anemia. He also had a large referral practice in rheumatic diseases, because he was an enthusiastic therapist and most physicians preferred to avoid the peculiar problems of arthritic patients. Dynamic, dogmatic, sometimes domineering, and brilliant, he was the very essence of good manners in clinical practice, treating equally those of high and low estate.[3] A superb clinician, he impressed both patients and physicians by the speed at which he arrived at correct conclusions. His first appointment to the staff was Dr. A. Carlton Ernstene as head of the Department of Cardiorespiratory Disease in

1932. Ernstene was trained in internal medicine and cardiology on the Harvard services of Boston City Hospital and was on the Harvard faculty. He had interests in laboratory and clinical research and was an excellent choice to direct the new department. Small departments of gastroenterology, allergy, and physical medicine were established during the next five years and, except for adding a few staff members, no further growth occurred before World War II. Economic restrictions imposed by the great depression required the staff to devote most of their energy to patient care, provided in large volume at low cost. Dr. H. S. Van Ordstrand joined Ernstene as a colleague in that department in 1939, heading a section of pulmonary disease.

With a gradually improving economy there were visions of expansion, only to be dimmed by World War II. Young physicians who might have been added to the staff were taken into the military services. This happened to several members of the staff in the medical division. The entire cardiorespiratory department was depleted by the departures of Ernstene and Van Ordstrand. Dr. Fay A. LeFevre, a former fellow, returned to the Clinic to replace them. Military needs also reduced the number of resident physicians in the training program. Immediately after the war there was a rapid increase in the number of the staff and further specialization. Young physicians realized the value of group practice as a result of their military experience, and many of them applied for training. Haden preferred to accept any physician who had served his country and actually accepted for training more than the teaching program needed.

Haden retired in 1949, and the mantle of chairman of the medical division fell on Ernstene. Aside from his love of work and clinical ability, he had little in common with Haden. Small in stature, he was handsome and personable in a quiet way. Meticulous order was his hallmark. He started his hospital rounds at 8 A.M. and finished in one hour. He might complete some brief unscheduled activities rapidly before returning to his office, by which time he expected his first patient of the day to have been examined by his resident. He would question the patient closely, recheck much of the physical examination, and make careful and concise notes in a small, tight, even script. Although he had a good background in internal medicine, cardiology was his field, and he had all the attributes of an outstanding clinical cardiologist.[4]

Seven new departments were established during Ernstene's tenure as chairman of the Division of Medicine,[5] and the Department of Cardiorespiratory Disease was divided into two departments, clinical cardiology and pulmonary disease. Administrative duties became heavy for one engaged in a large practice and serving as president or officer of several national medical societies. A representative Medical Committee was formed to advise and assist him, and this was the beginning of a democratic Division of Medicine. The chairman became the head of a committee of elected members of the division.

Ernstene retired as chairman in 1965 and was succeeded by Van Ordstrand, his first colleague in the old Department of Cardiorespiratory Disease. Expansion of the division continued under the successive chairmanships of Van Ordstrand and Drs. Ray A. Van Ommen and Richard G. Farmer. These three were specialists in pulmonary disease, infectious disease, and gastroenterology, respectively; but none had a provincial interest in his own department and each sought a balanced development of the division. In 1921, Phillips, Tucker, and Henry John were the entire staff of the division; in 1932 the staff consisted of eight members; in the next decade, the number increased to 15; and when Dr. Haden retired the number stood at 28. By 1969 the division had increased to 65 members, and in 1984 there were 141 staff members in the Division of Medicine.

Dr. Crile was interested in blood pressure all his professional life and early in his career made notable contributions to the knowledge of maintenance of blood pressure under certain conditions. Through the years he became convinced that hypertension was mediated through the sympathetic nervous system and that denervation of the celiac ganglion of that system would be beneficial to the hypertensive patient. He did a considerable amount of experimental and clinical work in this field. Although the therapeutic results of his surgical endeavors did not meet his expectations, he remained interested in hypertension and tried, with mixed success, to interest others of the staff.

In time, drugs for the effective treatment of high blood pressure became available. Many of them received early clinical testing at the Clinic, and a great many patients were referred for treatment of hypertension. Life and relative comfort could be prolonged even when kidney function was seriously impaired as a result of hypertension or other conditions. Dr. Willem J. Kolff developed the artificial kidney in Holland at the end of World War II and demonstrated its utility in the treatment of reversible kidney disease. Kolff came to the Clinic to start a Department of Artificial Organs shortly after the war. Eventually it was recognized that life could be prolonged greatly by regular dialysis in the absence of appreciable function of the kidneys. Urologic surgeons at the Clinic did a great deal of work on transplantation of kidneys taken from cadavers or relatives of the afflicted individual. Control of blood pressure, dialysis, and renal transplantation are still important therapeutic tools; the era of interest in hypertension at the Clinic started about 50 years ago and is still with us.

Kolff was one of a trio of physicians that influenced cardiology at the Clinic. The other two were Dr. F. Mason Sones, Jr. and Dr. Donald B. Effler, a cardiovascular surgeon. Kolff knew how to stop the heart and then to restore its beat, and Sones's diagnostic technics led the way to corrective cardiac surgery. There were times when these three men did not get along with one another. Even with mended relationships, the tensions never were fully resolved. Kolff left the Clinic in 1967 to continue his work with artificial organs at the University of Utah. Like Effler and Sones, his contributions during his Cleveland years were monumental and received international acclaim. Effler's and Sones's effect upon one another became so stressful—not only to them but to others around them—that by 1974 it required the intercession of the Board of Governors.[6]

In the late 1950s image-amplifying radiographic equipment became available, and Sones became interested in photographing the coronary arteries. Some incidental photographs showing portions of the coronary arteries had been made in Sweden earlier, but Sones made purposeful attempts to photograph the vessels, injecting contrast solution near the openings of the coronary arteries. A large dose was accidentally injected directly into a coronary artery. When no dire consequences were noted, Sones intentionally injected small doses of contrast material directly into the coronary arteries. As with Roentgen's discovery of x-rays, a brilliant insight turned an accident into a great advance. Thus began selective coronary arteriography, the first tremor of an earthquake whose reverberations are still rumbling. Soon Sones demonstrated that an artery implanted into heart muscle had formed connections with the coronary arteries, and so began the first effective coronary operation.[7] Coronary and other arteries are commonly affected by atherosclerosis, a form of "hardening of the arteries." Demand for coronary arteriography and the bypass operation soon developed and has persisted to this day.

Although the treatments of hypertension and coronary artery disease have greatly affected the growth of the institution, significant advances in clinical medicine have been initiated or popularized in many departments of the medical division. The first medical specialty in the Cleveland Clinic was endocrinology; Dr. Henry J. John set up the diabetic service in 1921. A formal Department of Endocrinology was instituted in 1928 with Dr. E. Perry McCullagh as head. McCullagh had started his training in surgery but gradually shifted his interest to endocrinology, a new subspecialty at the time. As is true in all new fields, the combination of intensive effort, keen insight, and investigative talent made him famous in his specialty. After John left the Clinic, McCullagh's interest in diabetes continued and soon included the entire field of endocrinology. He was a walking encyclopedia, a colorful and friendly person and an inexhaustible supplier of poems, jokes, and stories. Sometimes he gave orders vague to others but clear to himself. Once his resident misinterpreted a McCullagh order and requested that a radiologic examination of the colon be done on a woman who had no gastrointestinal symptoms. The patient was having the x-ray study when McCullagh was making rounds, and he was visibly annoyed. He castigated the resident for writing the order, stating that the order had been perfectly clear. The x-ray film showed a large cancer of the colon, and McCullagh accepted the report in good grace and with compliments to the resident.

In the early days McCullagh was engaged in laboratory and clinical research, especially with the hormones testosterone and intermedin, for which his work received wide recognition. He believed in rigid control of the blood glucose level of diabetics, an idea that was discounted later but now is being revived. McCullagh was also instrumental in founding Camp Ho-Mita-Koda, the oldest summer camp in the world for diabetic children. Diabetes has remained a primary interest of members of the department, headed successively by Dr. Penn G. Skillern and Dr. O. Peter Schumacher.

One of the first specialists appointed to the staff was Dr. Earl W. Netherton, head of the Department of Dermatology from 1923 to 1958. A treasured rotation of the residents in internal medicine was dermatology, a specialty omitted or disliked in most training programs at the time. Training under Netherton sharpened observational skills. He vividly described skin lesions in beautiful handwriting, ending with the diagnosis and treatment, each prescription being entered in full in the chart without abbreviations, even in the directions. Patients were to return for follow-up with the medications that were prescribed. Sometimes Netherton would rub ointments between his fingers, and occasionally would call the dispensing pharmacist to tell him that an ointment had not been prepared properly. He was a pioneer in dermatopathology and safe radiation therapy for skin diseases, and he was an expert in the tedious investigation of patients having contact dermatitis. In teaching he was kindly, saying after an inexperienced resident had made a ridiculous diagnosis, "Well, that's something to be considered but. . . ." He then would give a logical differential diagnosis. Dr. John R. Haserick succeeded Netherton as the head of dermatology in 1958. Haserick was best known for his contributions to the diagnosis and treatment of disseminated lupus erythematosus, a disease usually affecting the skin but also the general health that frequently resulted in death of the untreated patient. Haserick left the Clinic for an academic post, and Dr. Henry H. Roenigk, Jr. succeeded him as chairman in 1966. The present head of the department is Dr. Philip L. Bailin. In recent years new treatments for psoriasis and other diseases of the skin have been pioneered in the department, and laser beam therapy is used to treat several dermatologic diseases.

The Department of Cardiology had its roots in the Department of Cardiorespiratory Diseases, established in 1932 with Ernstene as head. Ernstene continued as head of that department, named Clinical Cardiology in 1960, at the time when the introduction of diagnostic laboratory studies led to the offshoot in that same year of the Department of Pediatric Cardiology. This latter department became the Department of Cardiovascular Disease and the Cardiac Laboratory in 1967. Sones was appointed head of this department. Sones made many technical and clinical advances. Ernstene retired in 1965 as head of the Department of Clinical Cardiology; Dr. William L. Proudfit succeeded him. Although the two departments of cardiology overlapped in many areas, their relationships were harmonious.[8]

A search committee was created to find a replacement for Proudfit, who had served past the usual age for retirement from administrative duties, and his successor would be chairman of a new Department of Cardiology, a merger of the Department of Clinical Cardiology and the Department of Cardiovascular Disease and the Cardiac Laboratory. Dr. William C. Sheldon became the chairman of the consolidated departments in 1975.[9] Sones continued his work in the cardiac laboratory.

Dr. E. N. Collins came to the Clinic as a radiologist in 1931. His interest in gastrointestinal radiology led him to specialize in disorders of the digestive tract. By 1934 his reputation was firmly established as "a stomach specialist," and he was asked to set up a Department of Gastroenterology. Collins thus became a practicing internist. With background in radiology and an aptitude for teaching, his service was popular with trainees. When he died in 1959, Dr. Charles H. Brown became head of the department. While Brown was directing the gastroenterology department, two important additions to the staff were made: Dr. Benjamin H. Sullivan, Jr. and Dr. Richard G. Farmer. Sullivan was a pioneer in the development and popularization of fiberoptic endoscopy, and his international influence greatly affected the practice of that specialty. Farmer, destined to succeed Brown as chairman of the department, shared Brown's interest in inflammatory bowel disease, and with his colleagues in pediatrics, surgery, and pathology Farmer led the Clinic to a worldwide reputation in the management of this troublesome affliction. Farmer now plays a key role in the leadership of the Clinic as chairman of the Division of Medicine, and his successor as department chairman is Dr. Bertram Fleshler. The department has 14 members, including a section of endoscopy, two pediatric gastroenterologists, and two members who also have appointments in the Division of Research.

The Department of Allergy was created in 1934 with Dr. I. M. Hinnant as head. Dr. Hinnant was followed successively as department head by Dr. J. Warrick Thomas, Dr. C. R. K. Johnston, and Dr. Richard R. Evans. Evans was co-discoverer of the definitive enzymatic defect responsible for a condition known as hereditary angioneurotic edema. The present head is Dr. Joseph F. Kelley. Kelley and two colleagues share the work of a busy department, emphasize diagnostic testing and treatment of allergy, and maintain a broad interest in internal medicine. Pediatric allergy is an area of particular interest in the department.

The need for a Department of Neuropsychiatry brought Professor Louis J. Karnosh from Western Reserve University to the Clinic. Dr. Karnosh's stature in his field lent immediate prestige to the new department. His colleagues said that what he did not know about the current state of neuropsychiatry was either unimportant or false. Karnosh was a master neuropsychiatrist who inspired the confidence of patients, residents, and colleagues. He had a stern countenance with sharp features, and his good sense of humor was intensified by his deadpan delivery of repartee. Of a plain background himself, he was not impressed by wealth or social position. Sharp insightful questioning and meticulous physical examination characterized his clinical approach. His questioning and therapeutic recommendations could be severe, but only when he thought severity was the best approach. Karnosh's clinical notes were a joy to read, not only because of artistic penmanship and precise use of the English language, but also because of what he wrote. So complete were his notes and so exquisitely phrased that he never dictated reports to physicians; his secretary merely copied his notes. Karnosh found time to give to his college and time to write books and illustrate them with superb woodcuts of his own making. He built a model railroad system and cultivated an encyclopedic knowledge of railroading. As a lecturer, he would capture the attention of his audience. Aware that he was uncommonly talented, he found it was unnecessary to announce the fact.

When Karnosh retired in 1960, Dr. Guy H. Williams, Jr. succeeded him as the new head of the department. Williams advised the separation of neuropsychiatry into two departments, and this was accomplished in 1967. Williams continued as head of the Department of Neurology. A gentle, good-humored, and accomplished physician, Williams was popular with the staff. He gradually expanded his new department and developed an outstanding section of electroencephalography.

As with other specialties, neurology became so complex that subspecialization was necessary for optimal patient care. The department grew in the 1970s and by 1984 there was a staff of 19. Dr.

John P. Conomy became department chairman in 1976, succeeding a brief but productive period of leadership by Dr. Arnold H. Greenhouse. Greenhouse's contribution was the recruitment of several able young neurologists, the vanguard of several other appointments to the staff over the following eight years as Conomy strengthened the department. Electrophysiology, cancer, epilepsy, neuromuscular disease, cerebrovascular disease, neuropathology, neuroradiology, neuro-otology, neuro-ophthalmology, and neurological research are among the several areas of specialization that the Clinic now supports in neurology and other departments. Much has happened since Karnosh began it all, nearly 40 years ago.

The new Department of Psychiatry with Dr. A. Dixon Weatherhead as head developed gradually. The addition of clinical psychologists and a section of child psychiatry were notable achievements. Dr. Richard M. Steinhilber became head of the department in 1977, sparking a five-year period of remarkable growth. Steinhilber built the department to number 13 psychiatrists. In addition, three clinical psychologists and one sociologist are members of the staff. Fields of interest and specialization include child and adolescent psychiatry, gender disorders, liaison psychiatry, disorders of eating, drug and alcohol addiction, chronic benign pain management, psychosexual disorders, biological psychiatry, and biofeedback. Growth and specialization are remarkable in this department, now a 17-year-old stepchild of neuropsychiatry. Steinhilber was succeeded by Dr. Neal Krupp.

The care of children in the Cleveland Clinic was not formalized in a Department of Pediatrics until 1951. By that time, increasing numbers of children came to the Clinic with rare or complicated diseases. The orientation of their treatment was disease centered, not child centered. But children are not simply small adults, and the arrival of Dr. Robert D. Mercer as head of the new department committed the Clinic to include a child-centered approach to the diagnosis and treatment of illness. In the 1920s, Phillips and Tucker, although not trained as pediatricians, had cared for many children in their large practices. Mercer was an assistant professor of pediatrics at Western Reserve University School of Medicine, well trained and with a fine reputation.

The increasing demand for pediatric consultation made it necessary to add another pediatrician almost immediately. A graduate medical training program in pediatrics was established, followed by undergraduate training of nurses in conjunction with the St. John School of Nursing and then by regular undergraduate teaching of medical students for the first time at the Foundation. The pediatricians provided care to the newborn following the establishment of a department of obstetrics.

The department's reputation was such that it joined in the work of every child-oriented facility in the community. Practice was heavily weighted toward neurologic disease, leukemia and other cancers, chronic diseases of the kidney, and congenital heart disease. Special interests were phenylketonuria, chromosome counting, and inflammatory disease of the bowel. Significant contributions have been made in the study of chromosomal abnormalities. Dr. Paul G. Dyment, succeeding Mercer as department chairman in 1979, joined the staff in 1971 as a pediatric cancer specialist. Dyment had joint appointments in the Department of Pediatrics and Department of Hematology and Medical Oncology. He was the first in a trend toward pediatricians with dual appointments. By 1984, the department had 15 members, 13 of them with joint appointments in Departments of Gastroenterology, Hematology and Medical Oncology, Cardiology, Hypertension and Nephrology, Neurology, Allergy, Endocrinology, Primary Care, and Gynecology. One member is jointly appointed in the Division of Anesthesiology with responsibility for pediatric intensive care. In ten of the 11 departments in the Division of Surgery are pediatric surgeons or surgeons giving much time to the care of children. With the exception of a gynecologist, the surgeons are not jointly appointed. As pediatrics advances, departmental lines become blurred. Specialty medicine shaped the organization of child care in the Clinic and led to the establishment of pediatrics. In other institutions, notably medical schools, the reverse has often been the case.

The Clinic formed the Department of Rheumatic Disease in 1953. Dr. Arthur L. Scherbel was the first chairman, serving for 27 years. In those days most practitioners felt discouraged when facing the problems of joint disease. Scherbel's optimistic attitude (in the tradition of Haden) helped to create a heavy demand for service.[10] Scherbel carried on alone until 1961. Important studies on cytotoxic drugs in rheumatoid arthritis, systemic lupus erythematosus, vasculitis, and allied disorders came from the department.[11] Dr. John

D. Clough succeeded Scherbel as department head. With the increasing clinical load and the developing interest of young physicians in the specialty, the department expanded under Clough's leadership to eleven physicians by 1984. Two of this number also have appointments in the Division of Laboratory Medicine. There are sections of clinical immunology, clinical pharmacology, special clinics, and clinical rheumatology. The Department of Physical Medicine and Rehabilitation was incorporated into the department as a section with Dr. Paul A. Nelson as head. In 1980, the name was changed to the Department of Rheumatic and Immunologic Disease.

Although Haden was primarily a hematologist, a Department of Hematology was not formed until 1953. Dr. John D. Battle was its first head. In the course of time, the medical treatment of cancer became another specialty, and the name was changed to the Department of Hematology and Medical Oncology. Dr. James S. Hewlett succeeded Battle in 1971, and when Hewlett retired as chairman, Dr. Robert B. Livingston led the department until 1982. Bone marrow transplantation, chemotherapy, and immunotherapy are among the treatments used by the staff in the department. Livingston established the predictive assay laboratory, where tumor cells from patients are grown and the effect of various chemotherapeutic agents on growth is determined. One of the important contributions of the department was Hewlett's use of exchange transfusion for effective treatment of a rare and almost always fatal disorder, thrombotic thrombocytopenic purpura. This treatment became the standard therapy until it was replaced by a much simpler technic of plasmapheresis, a method also pioneered at the Clinic. The members of the department have been active in testing experimental drugs or combinations of drugs in the treatment of malignant disease. This is a commitment requiring much time, accurate record keeping, careful analysis, and persistent optimism despite frequently discouraging responses. The search for effective new treatments continues, drawing upon the cooperation of all departments within the Clinic. Dr. James K. Weick succeeded Livingston as chairman in 1983.

Many patients are referred to the Department of Internal Medicine. The specialization of medical practice inevitably raised the question, is there a place for general internal medicine? Deciding in the affirmative, this department was formally established in 1949. John Tucker, its first chairman, had been a member of the Division of Medicine since 1921. He was succeeded by Dr. Leonard L. Lovshin. Dr. Ray A. Van Ommen became the third chairman. Van Ommen was also a chairman of the Division of Medicine and founded the Department of Infectious Disease. The ten physicians in this department have interests that include the whole field of internal medicine, and several are certified as subspecialists. The department is now headed by Dr. William H. Shafer, a gastroenterologist by training. Lovshin, now a member of the Emeritus staff, was well known for his interest in headaches.

For many years, mildly hypertensive patients were treated by general internists and cardiologists. Patients who had severe problems were studied in the hospital and then followed in the clinic by Dr. Robert D. Taylor, a member of the research department. As new drugs were available, it became evident that specialized service was required to supplement that provided by the Research Department. Dr. David C. Humphrey was appointed head of a new Department of Hypertension in 1959. Demands on the department increased and additional staff members were added. Dr. Ray W. Gifford, Jr. succeeded Humphrey as department head in 1967. One of the manifestations of kidney failure is severe hypertension, and kidney dialysis became a large clinical service, requiring much space and personnel. The dialysis program was moved into the Department of Hypertension and Nephrology from the research division. Members of the department have led in the development of two additional technics for the treatment of kidney failure: slow continuous ultrafiltration (SCUF) and continuous ambulatory peritoneal dialysis (CAPD). All these procedures prolong life in end-stage renal disease, but transplantation is more satisfactory when practical. The first cadaver kidney transplantation was done elsewhere, but in 1963, the Clinic was one of the first institutions to develop this advance in treatment. The department cooperates with the Department of Urology in the selection and treatment of patients in the transplantation program.

Hypertension secondary to renal artery disease has been the interest of members of this department along with others in the Department of Urology and in the Research and Radiology Divisions. Important advances in diagnosis and treatment have been made. The department consists of 14 members, and within the department special fields of interest include immunology, tissue typing, organ preservation, renal physiology, and pediatric kidney disease.

LeFevre spent two years as a fellow in medicine at the Clinic, followed by a year of postgraduate study in London and several years in practice in Cleveland before he joined the staff of the Clinic in 1942. He single-handedly maintained the Department of Cardiorespiratory Disease after the departures of Ernstene and Van Ordstrand for military service. With Ernstene's return and the addition of more staff in the department, LeFevre concentrated on his main interest, diseases of blood vessels, especially in the lower limbs. In 1952 he was appointed head of a new section, peripheral vascular disease. Dr. Victor G. deWolfe, who had had training in peripheral vascular disease in New York and had been a member of the staff since 1949, joined LeFevre. A separate Department of Peripheral Vascular Disease was formed in 1955. LeFevre was its head. When his duties as chairman of the Board of Governors encroached excessively on his time for practice, deWolfe succeeded him in 1961.

Dr. Jess R. Young is now chairman of this department, which works closely with the peripheral vascular surgeons. A clinical laboratory for study of patients with peripheral vascular disease was set up in 1977 by deWolfe. The diagnosis and treatment of peripheral vascular disease is not as formal in many institutions as it is at the Clinic. Teaching has been an important activity of the department.

The Department of Pulmonary Disease separated from the Department of Cardiorespiratory Disease in 1958. Van Ordstrand, who later became chairman of the Division of Medicine, was its first head. Van Ordstrand is known for his original description of acute berylliosis, a peculiar condition occurring in some workers exposed to beryllium. Dr. Joseph F. Tomashefski succeeded Van Ordstrand as department head. Tomashefski set up the pulmonary function laboratory. The five staff members have subspecialty interests in laboratory testing, fiberoptic bronchoscopy, respiratory therapy, environmental and occupational diseases of the chest, exercise physiology, malignant disease, and chronic obstructive pulmonary disease. Dr. Muzaffar Ahmad succeeded Tomashefski in 1983.

The Department of Infectious Disease had its origin as a section of infectious disease in the Department of Internal Medicine. Van Ommen was head of both the department and the section. In 1972 the section was made a separate department with Dr. Martin C. McHenry as head. The coincidence of a dynamic personality and a rapidly developing field was fortunate. McHenry has been active in studying the pharmacology and clinical use of several new antibiotics. Difficult infections of the heart, bloodstream, and bone have been the subjects of concentrated study. Many patients are referred to the Clinic with septic, terminally functioning kidneys. They have provided an opportunity for investigation of antibiotic treatment. In 1984 there were three staff members in the department.

In the late 1940s several corporations began to refer their executives for periodic physical examinations. Ernstene assigned staff physicians to examine individuals from specific companies. With expanding referral practices and with narrowing specialty interests of some of the staff, the need for a section of executive health was recognized. It was organized by Van Ordstrand when he was chairman of the medical division in 1971. Dr. Alfred M. Taylor, now retired, was appointed head of that section and has been succeeded by Dr. Richard Matzen. The section is now a department, and three full-time internists comprise its staff. Each year 3,200 to 3,500 examinations are done in what is now the Department of Preventive Medicine.

The Department of Primary Health Care was established in 1974. The tremendous growth of the Foundation mandated some form of organized health care of high quality for employees and their families. In some ways this is like an in-house health maintenance organization. At present it requires the full-time services of five internists, three part-time pediatricians, and three nurse practitioners. In addition, consultative services with any member of the medical staff are available. Dr. Gilbert Lowenthal, Jr. has been department chairman from its inception and has led its very successful development.

The Division of Medicine has played an important role in the dramatic changes of medical practice in America and the world since the days when the Clinic first opened its doors. Two major discoveries were announced about the time of the founding, the use of iodine for the treatment of toxic goiter and the discovery of insulin.[12] These advances not only changed medical practice of the day but also stimulated clinical and basic research in other areas. This research led to improved methods of diagnosis and treatment of many diseases, and at the same time increased the complexity of medicine. Methods of practice at the Clinic have changed since 1921, and practice is now more scientific. But the approach to the patient is the same. Consultations with a number of physicians may be required but ultimately one physician is responsible for each patient's care.

Division of Surgery

The original Clinic and Hospital buildings were paid for mainly by the income from thyroidectomies. Dr. Crile alone did more than 25,000.

In 1921 Dr. Henry Plummer of the Mayo Clinic had only recently shown that when patients with Graves' disease were given iodine, hyperthyroidism was partially controlled and thyroidectomy was relatively safe. There was, therefore, a backlog of patients who had had hyperthyroidism for many years and who for the first time were considered to be operable. In 1921, moreover, Marine's observations on the value of iodine in preventing the type of goiter that was endemic in the Midwest, and especially in the Great Lakes region, had not yet been acted on, with the result that huge nontoxic goiters were common. With the improvements in technic introduced mainly by Crile and the Mayos, thyroidectomy had suddenly become not only safe but almost fashionable. The vast backlog of goiters of all kinds resulted in an ever increasing number of thyroid operations. In 1927 the number reached its peak with 2700 operations on the thyroid, an average of ten each working day. The largest number that Crile performed in a single day was 35. However, the number of operations done was somewhat higher than the number of patients treated, for in those days it was the custom, in bad-risk patients, to do the operation in stages, first ligating the superior thyroid arteries, then removing one lobe, and at another hospitalization removing the remaining one.

The greatest danger in this period was thyroid crisis, a dramatic chain of events, still only partially understood, that was likely to occur when a patient with Graves' disease and severe hyperthy-roidism was subjected to a general anesthetic, an operation, or even when he experienced an infection or a bad fright. The pulse rate soared, the heart often fibrillated, the temperature rose rapidly to 105 or 106 degrees Fahrenheit, and the patient literally consumed himself in the fire of his own metabolism. Ice bags and oxygen tents sometimes helped. Transfusions were tried, without avail. Once initiated, the crisis tended to run its course, reaching its peak on the second night after operation, and then, if the patient survived, subsiding.

Crile believed that emotion, particularly fear, tended to trigger the crisis, and to prevent fear he had developed a system that came to be known as "stealing the thyroid." The patient would not be told when the operation was to take place. Every morning, breakfast was withheld and the nurse-anesthetist (Miss Lou Adams was the senior one at that time) would go to the patient's bedside and give a little nitrous oxide analgesia—just enough to make the patient a bit giddy and confused. On the morning of the operation, the routine was the same, except that the analgesia was a little deeper, so that the patient in his or her euphoria took little or no notice of the team that moved in. All the instruments for the operation were on tables with wheels. The neck was prepared with ether, iodine, and alcohol, and then draped. A floor nurse or the patient's special nurse stood on a chair behind the head of the bed and illuminated the operative field with a shaded light that she held on the end of a three-foot pole.[13]

Crile, having just finished an operation in a nearby room, would come down the hall at full speed, followed by a bewildered group of visiting surgeons. Miss Emmy Barr, the supervisor of the oper-ating room, having checked to see that everything was ready, would show Crile his fresh gown and gloves and lead him to the next patient's room. The resident who had prepared the patient's neck and infiltrated it with a large amount of 0.5 per cent Novocain would mutter a few words of the history. Crile would repeat these to the visitors with embellishments based on his philosophy about the kinetic system of man and animals. With a single stroke he would make a gracefully curved skin incision and then dissect the skin flap superficial to the platysma. He never stopped to clamp bleeders; that was the function of the first assistant. The second assistant, hanging uncomfortably over the framework of the head of the bed, was supposed to retract the skin and cut the thread after knots were tied. There was no conversation between the members of the team. Crile never asked for an instrument; he merely put out his hand and the instrument was slapped into it with a pop. All the while Crile would be talking to the visitors about everything from the patient's problems to the relations of the adrenal to hyperthyroidism and the relative size of the adrenals and brains of lions and alligators.

The operations were rapid, bloody, and unanatomic. In those days, before the advent of intravenous anesthesia, there was emphasis on speed. A transfusion team was always available to give blood when there was excessive loss. The same team stood ready to do tracheotomies when necessary, for in those days the incidence of injury to the recurrent laryngeal nerves was high.

Crile made no attempt either to ligate the inferior thyroid artery or to visualize the parathyroids or the nerve. In most cases there was enough of the gland left in the tracheoesophageal groove to protect the important structures, but when bleeding was excessive the hemostats sometimes overshot their mark and damaged the nerve. In recurrent goiters the incidence of injury to the nerve was very high. Postoperative hemorrhage was fairly common too, for the main vessels were not tied. Yet the organization was so superb that the mortality rate of the operations was the lowest that had ever been reported. For that reason, patients flocked to the Clinic from all over the world.

Operating with Crile was never a relaxing experience, nor was it always grim. He always noticed when there was a new second assistant and recognized him in a unique way, addressing himself to the first assistant. The moment the dialogue started, everyone except the neophyte leaning over the bedstead and trying desperately to cut the catgut knots knew what was coming.

"It must have rained last night," Crile would say to his assistant.

"Yes," would be the reply, "but how did you know?"

"Because the snails are out this morning," Crile would say, and there in the incision stood two sprigs of catgut, cut too long for Crile's taste, and looking for all the world like horns of snails.

From 1927 on, the incidence of thyroidectomy at the Cleveland Clinic declined steadily. With the advent of better anesthesia, better technic, and better surgical training, more and more thyroidectomies were done in the community hospitals. The introduction of iodized salt and the wider shipment of food from nonendemic to endemic areas resulted in a decreased incidence of nodular goiter. Next came antithyroid drugs and then radioactive iodine, making it no longer necessary to operate on patients for Graves' disease. Control of nodular goiter by feeding desiccated thyroid, the diagnosis of thyroiditis by needle biopsy and its treatment by corticosteroids or thyroid feeding, and the treatment of thyroid cysts by aspiration have made it unnecessary to operate on goiters unless they are large enough to cause pressure or to be of cosmetic importance, or unless they seem to be malignant. Thus in 1969 only 124 thyroidectomies were performed. Interestingly, in this same year there were 32 operations on the parathyroid, 19 of them for adenomas. What happened, one might ask, to the patients in 1927 who had hyperparathyroidism, for in that year not a single diagnosis of parathyroid hyperfunction was made.

The trend from thyroid surgery has continued. In the past ten years, needle biopsies have been done routinely on all goiters that in the past might have been treated surgically. In this way it has been possible to eliminate the possibility of malignancy in 90 per cent of the goiters. As a result of the use of needle biopsy in 1979, only 27 thyroid operations were done, 47 per cent of these for cancer. In the same year, as a result of better diagnosis and of the reputation in this field built up by Dr. Caldwell B. Esselstyn, Jr., there were 60 operations for hyperparathyroidism.

As the number of operations for goiter waned, that of cancer of the colon and rectum increased. Dr. Thomas E. Jones, an accomplished abdominal surgeon, had visited Mr. Miles, a surgeon in London, and had come back with the technic of the one-stage combined abdominoperineal resection, which he proceeded in his own right to develop to a fine art. Visitors came from everywhere to watch Jones do three or four combined operations in a morning, each taking less than an hour, at a time when it took most surgeons three or four hours to do one. On two occasions, he completed the operation in 33 minutes. Again it was a triumph of superb organization in which Mrs. Elizabeth Graber, in charge of Jones's operating room, would, practically single-handedly, turn the patient over and in a matter of seconds put the patient in a position for the perineal part of the operation.

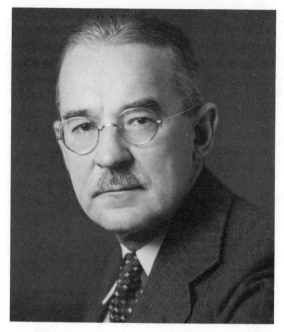

Thomas E. Jones, M.D.   Chief of Surgery, 1943–1949

Jones was operating in the days before sulfonamides or the antibiotics, and everywhere in the country at that time the mortality from colon resection with anastomosis was high. Peritonitis was the problem, but Jones avoided it by not opening the bowel or anastomosing it. Cancers that were located well above the rectum, even when they were frankly in the sigmoid, he would treat by combined abdominoperineal resection, establishing an end colostomy. After resections of the left colon or transverse colon, he almost never reestablished continuity by anastomosis, but exteriorized the tumor over a Rankin clamp, performing an obstructive resection. Thus, there were no anastomoses, except after resections of the right colon, and these, of course, were with the ileum and had few complications. The result was that Jones could report an astonishingly low mortality rate for surgery of the colon and rectum, although it was with a high incidence of colostomy, temporary or permanent.

Jones was a true general surgeon, whose versatility included not only abdominal surgery, but gynecology, varicose veins, radical dissections of the neck, and a limited amount of thoracic surgery. Several years before Dr. Evarts Graham of St. Louis reported his first successful pneumonectomy for cancer of the lung, Jones had performed a local resection of a lung cancer after which the patient lived for many years without recurrence. A pioneer in the use of radium and the gold radon seeds that were implanted into cancers, particularly in the oral cavity, Jones was a master of the technics of both radiation and surgery, and was in fact a leading authority on the treatment of cancer. Among other contributions, he was a pioneer in the use of a combination of electrocoagulation and implantation of radon seeds in selected low-lying rectal cancers. Although the results were excellent, he never reported them, perhaps because he was so satisfied with the combined abdominoperineal operation.

On September 29, 1949, when Jones was 57 years old and at the summit of his surgical career, he fell over while tying his shoe laces in the surgeons' locker room. Efforts at resuscitation failed, for he had been working all week with an occluded coronary artery, and an aneurysm of the left ventricle had ruptured. The Clinic suffered a severe blow, for at the time of his death Jones was carrying the main work load of the Department of General Surgery.

The other members of the department were Dr. Robert S. Dinsmore, long associated with Crile in thyroid and breast surgery, but without much interest in abdominal or other general surgical problems, and Dr. George Crile, Jr., who had trained under his father and Jones. Fortunately, Dr. Rupert B. Turnbull, Jr. had just finished his training with Jones. Jones had been grooming Turnbull to share with him the load of colon surgery. At the time of Jones's death, Turnbull had assisted in hundreds of operations on the colon but had performed only one by himself. It was a credit to Jones's ability as a teacher that in the next year Turnbull performed nearly a hundred operations on the colon, with a mortality rate as low as had been attained by Jones.

After Jones's death, Dinsmore became the administrative head of the Division of Surgery and head of the Department of General Surgery, titles be held until his illness and death in 1957. During that eight-year period, a large addition to the hospital was being built, and Dinsmore, with extraordinary forethought, planned the operating pavilion that is now named for him. Many members of the staff thought that the 23 operating rooms Dinsmore had planned were far too many for the Clinic's needs. Antibiotics were eliminating operations for infections, and antithyroid drugs and radio-

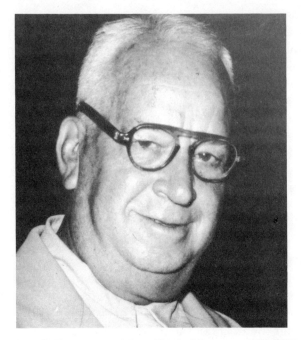

Robert S. Dinsmore, M.D.   Chief of Surgery, 1949–1957

active iodine were replacing surgery in the treatment of hyperthyroidism. But by the time the building was finished, the same antibiotics that eliminated one group of operations had made possible another and much larger group, so that from the first, the operating room space was fully occupied.[14] Ten years later it was found necessary to open six additional operating rooms to carry the ever increasing load of cardiac surgery.

By the time Dinsmore died, the system had changed, and the positions of autocratic division chiefs were abolished.[15] Dr. Stanley O. Hoerr, appointed to the staff of the Department of General Surgery shortly after Jones's death, and with considerable experience in administration at medical schools in Boston and Columbus, was appointed chairman of the Division of Surgery in 1957. At the same time, George Crile, Jr. became head of the Department of General Surgery. Thus, there arose an anomalous situation in which Hoerr was Crile's chairman in the division, and Crile, Jr. was Hoerr's in the department. Such an arrangement would be impossible in the hierarchies of many institutions, but because neither chief had an autonomous authority, and both needed the support of the various committees, the arrangement worked. It probably would have worked in any event, for both men were busy, respected one another, and had no cause for conflict.

Dr. James S. Krieger succeeded Hoerr as chairman of the Division of Surgery in 1971 and left office by reason of reaching the age of mandatory retirement from the position. Dr. Bruce H. Stewart, a urologic surgeon, served from 1980 until his death in 1983. Stewart's death created a most untimely loss. Dr. Ralph A. Straffon, Stewart's colleague and the chairman of the Department of Urology, was then appointed chairman of the Division of Surgery.

Hoerr's main interest was in surgery of the upper abdomen. Turnbull began to specialize in surgery of the large bowel, Humphries in vascular surgery, Effler in thoracic surgery, Krieger in gynecology, and Anderson in plastic surgery. Crile, Jr. continued to do general surgery, but as the years passed, limited himself increasingly to operations on the thyroid, upper abdomen and breast. Thus, the pattern of ultraspecialization that characterizes the Clinic continued to develop.

In 1968, Crile, Jr., who had always planned to retire, at least in part, at age 60, resigned as head of the Department of General Surgery and became a senior consultant. Hoerr served as head for one year and then he, too, at age 60 became a senior consultant. Dr. Robert E. Hermann, a member of the staff for several years with a special interest in teaching residents and interns, became head of the department. The most recent addition to the Department of General Surgery was a pediatric general surgeon. One surgeon has a special interest in parenteral nutrition.

From the professional standpoint, the contributions made by the Clinic's Department of General Surgery have been more of development than in the area of innovation. Jones was the great popularizer of the Miles operation; Hoerr did much to show the value of vagotomy and shunt operations; Crile, Jr. and Turnbull pioneered and popularized the radical surgical treatment of fulminating ulcerative colitis. Turnbull later introduced a diverting and drainage procedure which further lowered the mortality from this disease.

In the past 30 years the forces of conservatism have been at work. It is fair to say that in most of the surgical departments, and especially in general surgery, the main endeavor has been to find ways to avoid such morbidities as are associated with radical operations for cancer. Sphincter-saving operations for cancer of the rectum began to be employed much more often than the combined abdominoperineal resection. The low-anterior resection, especially when done with the modern stapler, enabled the surgeons to remove cancers and save the rectum. For small, low-lying cancers, especially if they were polypoid and protruded into the bowel, electrocoagulation or a special type of radiation treatment given through a proctoscope was used to destroy the tumor. As a result, in 1980 only 18 cancers of the rectum were treated by the radical operation that sacrificed the rectum and required a colostomy.

Modifications of radical cancer operations preserving muscles and nerves were advocated. In almost every field, including gynecology, in which Krieger staunchly defended the use of conization of the cervix over hysterectomy as the treatment for carcinoma in situ, the Clinic's surgeons adopted conservative technics and looked for ways to spare the patients radical operative treatment. In thoracic surgery, Effler preferred lobectomy to pneumonectomy whenever the smaller operation was feasible.

In 1955, Crile, Jr. began to treat selected patients with small cancers of the breast by wide local excision or partial mastectomy usually combined with axillary dissection. Radical mastectomy was abandoned, setting a trend that has become national. Later, in 1980, Esselstyn began to combine local excision of small breast cancers with specialized radiation given by Drs. Antunez and Jelden. At present, the breast is being saved in more than 60 per cent of the patients with cancer of the breast. Most of the development was during a period in which the national and worldwide swing was towards ever more prophylactic, more extensive and more deforming operations. In recent years, however, the Clinic's conservative philosophy of treatment has gained wide acceptance.

Urology and ear, nose, and throat were the only surgical specialties represented when the Clinic opened. At that time, urology was not completely separated from general surgery, for during the early years Lower performed almost as many thyroidectomies, cholecystectomies, and a variety of general surgical operations as urologic procedures. However, Dr. Justin M. Waugh, an ear, nose, and throat surgeon, stayed close to his specialty, and when orthopedic surgery, neurological surgery, and ophthalmology were introduced,

Dickson and Locke and Ruedemann were strictly specialized in their respective fields. The same applied to the other specialties, plastic surgery, gynecology, thoracic surgery, vascular surgery, and colorectal surgery as they became differentiated from general surgery. General surgery then remained as one of the smaller specialty services and was limited essentially to the treatment of diseases of the upper abdomen, thyroid, and breast, and to the repair of hernias. It is interesting to consider, in more detail, the changes in the type of practice that have taken place in the specialties since they were introduced.

In 1921, tonsils and adenoids were the preoccupation of the ear, nose, and throat surgeon. The concept of chronic infection as a cause of man's ills, from arthritis to ulcer, was gaining in popularity, and the tonsils bore the brunt of the surgeon's assault. In those days, too, before sulfanilamide and antibiotics, the greatest challenge to the otologist was the treatment of infections of the mastoid. Corrections of deviated nasal septa were also in vogue, but at that time nothing could be done surgically to help deafness. If cancers and papillomas of the larynx were common, it did not appear so from the Clinic's operative schedules, but that was before the increasing use of cigarettes had had time to produce results.

After Waugh's retirement, Dr. William V. Mullin carried on and did much to develop the technic of operations on the mastoid. After Mullin's untimely death from an overwhelming bacterial infection, Dr. Paul M. Moore headed the department, later resigning in favor of Dr. Harold E. Harris, a young surgeon with superb technical skill and clinical judgment. By that time, it was the 1940s, and cancers of the larynx were becoming common. Pediatricians and internists were beginning to take a second look at tonsillectomy and to wonder whether the tonsils did not perhaps serve some useful immunologic function. But most important, Lempert had shown the feasibility of operating for otosclerosis, a disease that fused together the tiny bones of the inner ear and caused progressive deafness. He was scoffed at by many, but his patients recovered their hearing. He organized a course to teach other otolaryngologists how to do it. Harris was among the first to apply.

When Harris requested approval of the chief of the Division of Surgery to attend the course, the request was refused, but he attended it anyway. By the time he returned, the Administrative Board had investigated and decided that Harris had been right, and they refunded his expenses and the tuition that he had paid.

As a result of being one of the first to learn the new technic of the operation on the stapes, Harris was swamped with patients requiring operations for otosclerosis. By 1955, the operations in which Harris had been trained in his residency (i.e., tonsillectomy, adenoidectomy, mastoidectomy, and correction of deviated septum) had all but disappeared from the schedules. In their place were the new operations on the inner ear and operations for cancers of the larynx, tongue, and mouth. The care of patients with these cancers caused conflict with the newly formed Department of Plastic Surgery. Bronchoscopic examinations, historically in the field of the laryngologists who first developed the technic, were rapidly falling into the province of the thoracic surgeons who were the ones who would operate on whatever pulmonary disease was visualized. Thus, there was a struggle among these three departments. The struggle could not be resolved by tradition, because there was no tradition. Some ear, nose, and throat surgeons performed radical neck dissections for cancers of the mouth and larynx, and others confined themselves to the treatment of the primary tumors. In some institutions, the ear, nose, and throat surgeons did all the bronchoscopies and the general surgeons performed the chest operations, whereas in other institutions the thoracic surgeons performed both bronchoscopy and chest surgery. Resolution of the problem associated with this type of overlap between departments seemed insolvable, and at that time it probably could not be resolved without the loss of one or more of the able surgeons who were vying with one another for what they considered to be their turf.

If there had been an authoritarian chief of surgery, empowered to make an arbitrary decision, the Clinic might have suffered a serious loss. As it was, the Surgical Committee, composed of the contestants' knowledgeable peers, acted discreetly and with tact. They took no action on the bronchoscopy issue, believing that there would be enough bronchoscopies to provide training for residents in both departments. In respect to the neck dissection dispute, they appointed a subcommittee that was empowered to review the results of all neck dissections in the presence of the surgeons who had done them. It soon became clear to all concerned that surgeons in the

Department of Plastic Surgery, who had been trained in their residencies to perform radical surgery, performed the operations in about a third the time and with fewer complications than did those whose training had been primarily in the treatment of the primary tumor. Soon the plastic surgeons and the otolaryngologists were cooperating, the latter doing the laryngeal part of the operations and the plastic surgeons performing the neck dissections, assisted by the otolaryngology residents. A major conflict had been resolved without loss of face, loss of excellence, or loss of surgeons.

Since the death of Harris and his replacement by Dr. Harvey M. Tucker as chairman, the Department of Otolaryngology and Communicative Disorders has continued to grow and subspecialize. There are now six members of the department. Cancer of the head and neck, reconstruction of nerves (such as facial and inferior laryngeal), cosmetic surgery of the face, and problems related to hearing are areas of special interest. On the diagnostic side there are many intricate tests of hearing, including one called "brain-stem evoked auditory response" in which a series of blips is sounded in the ear. These impulses stimulate electrical waves in the brain that can be isolated and studied. There is also a vestibular physiologist interested in the diagnosis and treatment of dizziness. Otolaryngology has come a long way since the days when it was devoted chiefly to the removal of tonsils and adenoids.

Since the recruitment of a group of otolaryngologists with special interests and training in cancer, much of the radical treatment of cancers of the neck formerly referred to the Department of Plastic Surgery is done in the Department of Otolaryngology and Communicative Disorders.

Conficts similar to the above arose between neurological and orthopedic surgery in respect to which department should be responsible for surgery of the intervertebral disks, and between thoracic surgery and general surgery over the question of who would operate on diverticula of the pharynx and cancers of the lower esophagus and the upper stomach. In each case the problem was solved by a review of the results of surgery. When there was no difference in the results, no action was taken. When there was a difference, no legislation was passed, but the differences were made known and in time most of the operations were referred to the surgeons who had the best results. On one occasion, equally good results from treating the same disease in two departments were reported in a jointly authored paper.

From the time the Department of Neurological Surgery was established by Locke in 1924, it was a strong one. After Locke's death in the disaster, Dr. W. James Gardner came from Philadelphia to be head of the department. Gardner's long and brilliant career combined superlative skill and a genius for innovation. Associated with him for 30 years was Dr. Alexander T. Bunts, son of the founder, who emphasized the surgical treatment of protruded intervertebral disks and spinal cord tumors.

Gardner's inventiveness and his many contributions to the art and philosophy of neurologic surgery have given him a special place among the world's great neurosurgeons. He developed the pneumatic suit to maintain blood pressure or control bleeding (an adaptation of Crile's early work), the alternating air pressure mattress for prevention of bed sores, and the pneumatic splint for fractures. After Gardner's retirement, Dr. Wallace B. Hamby succeeded him. Hamby had trained under Gardner and had developed a national reputation for his work in the diagnosis and treatment of aneurysms of the arteries of the brain. He in turn was succeeded by Dr. Donald F. Dohn, whose department continued to show leadership in neurologic surgery, including proficiency in the stereotactic operation for control of the symptoms of Parkinson's disease, and the destruction of the pituitary by implanting radioactive yttrium. After Dohn left the Clinic, Dr. Joseph F. Hahn became department chairman. At present there are four members of this department, one with a special interest in pediatric neurosurgery and epilepsy, another concerned with cerebrovascular problems and bypass operations, a third whose work is largely confined to the treatment of problems of the spine, and a fourth who specializes in cancers of the brain and spinal cord.

Orthopedic surgery, introduced as a specialty in 1922, was under the direction of Dr. James A. Dickson, a surgeon of great originality and an internationally recognized leader in his field. Before it became common practice to insert metal hip joints, Dickson had perfected an elegant operation called geometric osteotomy, in which an unhealed fracture of the hip was rotated to promote healing. During his tenure, which lasted until 1954 when he was succeeded by Dr. James I. Kendrick, he witnessed the decline and fall of osteomyelitis as a major orthopedic problem, and the development of artificial joints and a number of operations designed to correct arthritis. Again, in orthopedic surgery the types of operations done today are entirely different from those done in the 1920s. Scoliosis, for example, is now often treated by internal fixation, the vertebrae being held in place by a metal prosthesis resembling a jack. Dr. Charles M. Evarts, succeeding Kendrick as chairman of the Department of Orthopedic Surgery, was one of the first to popularize this form of treatment. A successful sports medicine department was introduced under Dr. H. Royer Collins. This section now utilizes four physicians and an exercise physiologist. Collins followed Evarts as chairman. In 1984, the Orthopedic Department, headed by Dr. Alan H. Wilde, had a total staff of 17 men. Replacement of joints, hand surgery, pediatric orthopedics, treatment of curvature of the spine, orthopedic oncology (tumors of the bone), and disorders of the back are among the subspecialties in the department. One member of the department is a medical orthopedist concerned with diagnosis and medical treatment, and one is a podiatrist. One of the commonest operations done by the Clinic's orthopedists is replacement of joints. More than 500 of these operations were done in 1983, chiefly hips and an increasing number of knees and shoulders and some ankles. Much surgery is also done on the joints of arthritic fingers. Subspecialization has been the key to the orthopedic department's success.

There is perhaps no field of surgery in which the march of science had made such profound changes as in urology. In the 1920s, before sulfanilamide, the treatment of gonorrhea was one of the urologist's main occupations. Suprapubic prostatectomy was another. Then came transurethral resection of the prostate and of bladder tumors, and a whole new set of technics had to be learned. Dr. William J. Engel, urologist and son-in-law of Dr. Lower, was a master of the transurethral resectoscope. Dr. Charles C. Higgins, who succeeded Lower as head of the Department of Urology, became famous for his "acid ash diet," a sometimes successful means of dissolving, but mainly an effective way of preventing, the growth of kidney stones. He was also a pioneer in the development of the operation to transplant into the lower bowel the ureters of children with exstrophy of the bladder. He operated on the world's largest series of these patients, and had one of the world's largest series of cystectomies for cancer of the bladder.

In 1934 Dr. Harry Goldblatt, a Cleveland pathologist, discovered that partial blockage of a renal artery was a cause of hypertension. Acting on this, Dr. Eugene F. Poutasse soon developed the technic of renal arteriography and discovered that in a large number of patients renal hypertension could be corrected by removing the obstruction, grafting in a new vessel, or removing the part of the kidney which the diseased artery supplied.

After Higgins and Engel retired, Dr. Ralph A. Straffon became head of the department. In collaboration with Kolff, inventor of the artificial kidney and head of the newly formed Department of Artificial Organs, he initiated a kidney transplant program in which within a few years there were more successful transplantations of kidneys taken from cadaver donors than in any other reported series. In conjunction with the renal transplant program is a larger dialysis program, and also a tissue-typing laboratory which acts as a center for all tissue typing in northern Ohio. During recent years, the Cleveland Clinic group has established for the first time a classification of the different types of renovascular disease and has found that each lesion has a distinctive radiographic pattern, occurs in its own clinical setting, and has a different natural history when observed over a period of years. Basic knowledge of renovascular disease has been accumulated by close cooperation among the Department of Hypertension and Nephrology, the Department of Urology, and the Divisions of Radiology, Research, and Laboratory Medicine. Some patients with certain renovascular lesions may be safely followed under conservative treatment, thus allowing better selection of other patients for surgery, which in turn has improved the long-term operative results.

During 60 years, urologic practice has not only changed from the treatment of gonorrhea to the treatment of hypertension and renal failure, but the technics and scope of operations have evolved into something quite different. Instead of approaching the kidneys or adrenals through the back, the urologists now use an abdominal approach obtaining much better exposure and control of the vessels. They also are adept, often in cooperation with the Department of Colorectal Surgery, in implanting the ureters into isolated loops of intestine that are brought to the skin, for drainage, in patients whose bladders have been removed. In short, urology has emerged from a specialty devoted to medical practice and minor surgery to a major surgical specialty.

At the present time there are six staff urologists. Urological oncology, pediatric urology, transplantation, infertility, and impotence are subspecialties within the department.

Ophthalmology, a hybrid medico-surgical specialty, was introduced in 1924 under Dr. A. D. Ruedemann, a dynamic personality and capable surgeon. He acquired an enormous following, using a great deal of paramedical help in his office work, and seeing daily an extraordinarily large number of patients. In 1947, Ruedemann, always an independent worker and thinker, left the Clinic to accept a post at Wayne University.[16] He was succeeded by Dr. Roscoe J. Kennedy, who carried a heavy clinical load with distinction. Kennedy retired in 1969, and Dr. Froncie A. Gutman was appointed chairman of the Department of Ophthalmology. Between 1970 and 1983, the ophthalmology staff increased from a full time complement of two ophthalmologists to a full time staff of eleven ophthalmologists and one optometrist. In addition, the paramedical and technical staff of the department included approximately 60 people by 1984. Growth of the department was directed along subspecialty interests. Rapidly advancing technology impacted upon both the medical and surgical management of disease. Major breakthroughs included the use of the operating microscope, laser technology, vitrectomy surgery, intraocular lenses, and ocular ultrasonography.

Two ophthalmologists are interested primarily in corneal and external disease of the eye. Half of the cataract operations being done today are followed by a lens implant. Another ophthalmologist is interested in plastic procedures on the eye such as correction of eyelid deformities or treatment of cancer of the lids. Four members of the department treat retinal disease. There are two pediatric ophthalmologists who treat many children with crossed eyes, and there is a neuro-ophthalmologist concerned with neurological conditions that affect the eye. The optometrist is primarily a refractionist, prescribing corrective lenses for patients.

Gynecology was introduced as a specialty in 1950 under the leadership of Dr. James S. Krieger. Krieger came to the Clinic about the same time that the Papanicolaou smear became popular. He was interested in the conservative treatment of in situ carcinoma of the cervix by conization. While the rest of the country's gynecologists were debating whether the condition should be treated by radical or conservative hysterectomy with or without radiation, Krieger collected data to show that simple conization, almost an office procedure, was as effective as the more complex procedures, provided only that the status of the patient was followed thereafter by annual Papanicolaou tests. At first the object of bitter criticism, the concept gained popular support. After Krieger's retirement, the Department of Gynecology was taken over by Dr. Lester A. Ballard, Jr. The staff has increased to seven. At present there are two general gynecologists, two who are interested in gynecological malignancies, one who is interested in children and adolescents, and one who specializes in infertility and microsurgery.

Plastic surgery is one of the youngest surgical specialties in America, and the first formal training program in the specialty was established just a few years before World War II. Wounded soldiers in World War I who had recovered with serious deformities challenged surgeons in the 1920s and 1930s to become expert in technics of reconstruction and repair. Many of these surgeons had different backgrounds in training, and the emerging specialty was a hybrid of surgeons.

Dr. Robin Anderson, a general surgeon, was trained in St. Louis by some of the great American pioneers in plastic surgery. Stanley Hoerr had known Anderson for a number of years. Hoerr saw the need to develop plastic surgery at the Clinic, and Anderson accepted an invitation to join the Department of General Surgery in 1951. By the 1960s there were two full-time plastic surgeons in a separate department split off from general surgery. Anderson was chairman.

When Anderson retired in 1979, Dr. Melvyn I. Dinner became chairman, and a move into more spacious facilities permitted much needed growth of the department. Dinner recognized the importance of developing subspecialties within plastic surgery, and he encouraged that craniofacial, pediatric, hand, and microvascular technics be developed. In 1982, a section of maxillofacial prosthetics and dentistry was established within the department, providing support for the treatment and rehabilitation of patients with head and neck cancer and for patients with deformities of the jaws, face, and skull.

Dr. Salvatore J. Esposito is head of the dental section that now numbers two prosthetists, an oral surgeon, and a general dentist. At one time years earlier, there was a dental department in the Clinic, but it never became strong. The dentists on the staff investigated the general condition of patients' teeth insofar as other medical and diagnostic problems might be related to dental pathology, and much of the old dental treatment was extractions. Dr. Charles A. Resch was the last of the old department, and when he died in 1964 there was no replacement for him. Outside dental consultants, working at the Clinic a few hours per week, provided such services as were then desired by the medical staff.

Dinner left the Clinic in 1983 to enter private practice, and Dr. Shattuck W. Hartwell, Jr., a long-time member of the department and for many years the director of Professional Staff Affairs, accepted the request of the Board of Governors to be acting chairman in addition to his other duties while a search committee looked for a new chairman. The department now numbers six plastic surgeons and four dentists, and Hartwell continues to develop the subspecialty services that Dinner established.

The Department of Vascular Surgery, one of the first if not the first in this country, was started officially in 1957. It had been in operation as a subspecialty. In 1952 Crile, Jr. had gone abroad on a clinical tour, as every staff member had a chance to do, to determine what was going on in his field. He visited Mr. Charles Robb, a surgeon at St. Mary's Hospital in London, and there he saw the world's first artery bank. Impressed with the success of replacing a diseased artery with one from the bank, on his return to the Clinic Crile, Jr. discussed this with Dinsmore, and they decided that someone should be selected for this field. Since it was mainly the vessels of the lower extremity which were to be grafted, they decided to engage an orthopedist who would be able to do a good job of amputating the leg if and when the graft failed! Dr. Alfred W. Humphries, a junior member in the Department of Orthopedic Surgery, was tapped for the specialty, and within a year he was working fulltime at it. His skill as an amputator was rarely needed. He was the first surgeon in the area to have an artery bank; then he promoted the use of plastic grafts, and through the years he had great success in the treatment of all types of aneurysms. With the assistance of Dr. John Homi, then in the Department of Anesthesiology, a technic was devised to increase blood flow to the brain by having the patient inhale carbon dioxide, thus making possible operations on the carotid artery that previously had often led to brain damage from anoxia. Humphries and Dr. Edwin G. Beven performed between 800 and 900 operations on major blood vessels each year. Since Humphries' retirement, Beven (now chairman) and two associates continue to make progress in this difficult and demanding field.

As already mentioned, Turnbull took over much of the colon surgery after Jones's death. Before long he was doing it so well and was so expert in diagnosis and management that he was performing almost all of the operations. A Department of Colorectal Surgery was formed. Turnbull introduced many innovations and promoted many operations that avoid permanent colostomy and reduce morbidity. Dr. Victor W. Fazio succeeded Turnbull as chairman, and the department now has four full-time colorectal surgeons, one with a special interest in the colorectal diseases of children.

Among the diseases that are most commonly treated by the colorectal surgeons are the inflammatory diseases of bowel, ulcerative colitis, and Crohn's disease. Whether the hundred or more operations a year that are being done at the Clinic for these diseases is the result of the surgeons' reputations in a field that is so fraught with difficulties that many general surgeons try to avoid it, or whether it represents a true increase in the incidence of the disease, it is impossible to say. Perhaps the increased use of injections for immunization or treatments is causing autoimmunity and an attack by the immune system on the colon. In any event these diseases, which were so rare as to be a curiosity when Jones was operating in the 1930s, are now the most common serious diseases of the bowel seen at the Clinic.

The growth of cardiac surgery has been one of the most dramatic developments in the history of the Clinic. In 1948, Dr. Donald B. Effler became head of the Department of Thoracic Surgery. It seemed that the expanding new field was to be the treatment of cancers of the lung and the esophagus. A decade before, lung cancers had been considered rare, for the epidemic had not yet begun. At that time thoracic surgery consisted mainly of thoracoplasties for tuberculosis and draining empyemas and lung abscesses. Then when penicillin controlled pneumonia, and streptomycin made thoracoplasties less frequently necessary in the treatment of tuberculosis, the need for surgery in the treatment of these diseases all but vanished. But the rising incidence of lung cancer, first treated by total pneumonectomy in 1932 by Dr. Evarts Graham of St. Louis, soon

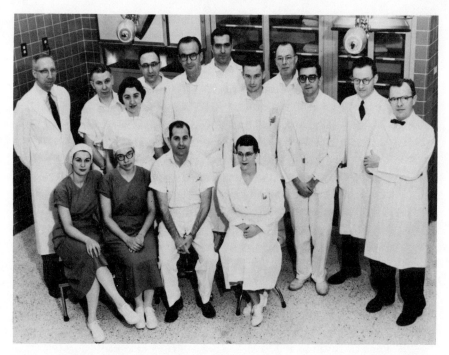

Leaders in the treatment of coronary artery disease. Standing: Willem J. Kolff, M.D., Artificial Organs (far left). Donald B. Effler, M.D., Thoracic and Cardiovascular Surgery (5th from left). Laurence K. Groves, M.D., Thoracic and Cardiovascular Surgery (6th from left). Donald E. Hale, M.D., Anesthesiology (4th from right). F. Mason Sones, Jr., M.D., Cardiology (far right). (photographed in 1956)

filled the gap. Then came the pioneering work of Dr. Robert Gross (in Boston) and Dr. John Jones (a California surgeon and brother of Thomas E. Jones), who began to ligate the ductus arteriosus. This was followed rapidly (in Baltimore) by Dr. Alfred Blalock's operation for the blue babies, and by the operation for mitral stenosis, a cardiac defect caused by rheumatic fever. Cardiac surgery thus began, but these were only the beginnings.

The Clinic's thoracic surgeons were poised to participate in the development of heart surgery. Some cardiac or vascular defects could be corrected or improved by relatively simple operations, but many would require a heart-lung machine to maintain the circulation during operation. Such machines were being developed, but the units were large and cumbersome and required a great deal of attention. Kolff, in the Department of Artificial Organs, constructed a mem-

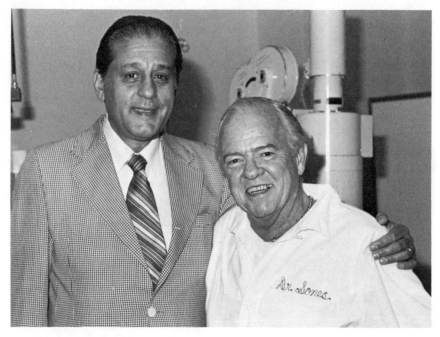

Drs. René G. Favaloro and F. Mason Sones, Jr.   (photographed in 1982)

brane oxygenator that was satisfactory for children not requiring a large volume of blood to be pumped. This permitted open-heart operations to be performed. Soon the machines were improved, increasing the latitude of relatively safe operations. But many problems remained. Kolff did animal experiments in which the heart's action had been temporarily arrested by injecting a solution of potassium into the coronary arteries. This technic was adapted for clinical use. Open-heart surgery was now a reality, but its development was not uneventful in the early days. Congenital and rheumatic valvular defects could be corrected with increasing frequency, and soon prosthetic valves could be inserted in the heart.

With Sones's demonstration that an internal mammary artery implanted in the heart muscle could form connections with the coronary arteries, there was great demand for this operation. A new era was born when, in occasional cases, a narrowed portion of a coronary artery could be excised and a vein inserted or the narrowed area slit lengthwise and a tapered gusset inserted to widen the narrowed portion, both procedures being followed by increased coronary blood flow. In May 1967, Dr. René Favaloro, an Argentine-born and Argentine-educated surgeon who was appointed to the Clinic staff after completing his training in thoracic and cardiovascular surgery, performed a bypass operation using the saphenous vein, thereby making history. Rapidly it was shown that the saphenous vein graft usually remained open, and symptoms were relieved. Operative mortality was low from the start and decreased further with time. Since 1971, the overall operative mortality for bypass surgery on a nonemergency basis and without valvular heart disease or other serious complications has been less than 1 per cent. There has been a tremendous demand for bypass surgery because of the relief of symptoms and improved survival. This demand along with the need for other operations on the heart and lungs results in heavy clinical loads for the seven cardiovascular surgeons on the staff at present. In 1983, 3,461 operations were performed on the heart, in addition to 325 major thoracic operations not involving the heart.

Favaloro returned to his homeland in 1971, where he remains an internationally acclaimed surgeon. Effler retired early to a more relaxed practice in 1975 and was succeeded by Dr. Floyd D. Loop as head of the department.[17] Loop has supervised the development of the department, improved operative technics, conducted extensive follow-up studies on patients who have had bypass operations, and sought means to control the costs of operative treatment. The use of an artery taken from the inside of the chest wall as a bypass vessel has been a major advance. Formerly, a great deal of blood was transfused into patients who had bypass operations, but now the average amount of blood used is two pints and 60 per cent of patients receive no blood.

Although operations for congenital heart disease were performed early in the department's history, there was a long interval of de-emphasis on congenital heart disease. The treatment of acquired heart disease commanded the most attention. Now there has been a resurgence of referrals for study and operative treatment of congenital heart disease following the appointment to the staff of a pediatric cardiologist and a pediatric cardiac surgeon. One surgeon in the department has been active in the artificial heart program in animals and in the temporary assist of the circulation by an artificial device in patients.

When one views the developments in surgery over the past 60

years, it is apparent that the Clinic's surgeons have been quick to exploit innovations. Emphasis has been more on development than on innovation, but in relation to their number, the Clinic's surgeons have contributed more than their share of innovations, too. Some surgeons have shown how medical or office treatment could supplant operations that before had been thought necessary. The ability to think in these terms, to view the practice of surgery not as a means of doing operations but as a way of giving effective treatment, whether medical or surgical, is encouraged by the fact that there is no incentive for the Clinic surgeons to perform a large number of operations. The salaries of the surgeons depend more on the scientific quality of the work in the estimate of their peers than on the dollars that patients pay for their services. It is helpful, too, to have access to the research facilities offered by the Clinic, and to have the cooperation of the skillful professionals who spend full-time in research. It seems, therefore, that the traditions of innovation and development initiated so many years ago by Bunts, by Lower, and particularly by Crile have been continued in an environment well suited to the study of clinical problems and to the discovery of their solutions in both the operating room and the laboratory.

Division of Anesthesiology

From 1921 to 1946, nurses administered anesthetics to patients. They dropped ether into gauzes laid over patients' airways or they used chloroform to "put them under." The nurses were responsible to the surgeon.

Physicians began to specialize in anesthesiology before World War II when new anesthetic agents and technics were being introduced.[18] The Clinic established a Department of Anesthesiology in the Division of Surgery after the war, and Dr. Donald E. Hale was chosen to be its head.

Hale had been a board-certified surgeon before developing an interest in anesthesiology, and he became certified in that specialty as well. With such a background, he was intellectually and psychologically equipped to understand the problems of dealing with surgeons and nurse anesthetists. Calm, kind, and good humored, Hale quickly gained the confidence of surgeons and internists. He was interested in clinical medicine, surgery, and research. When others were emotional under tense conditions, he appeared placid. There was a time when a serious complication beset a patient during an operation. The surgeon repeatedly instructed Hale relative to the administration of the anesthetic and blamed him without reason for the complications. In this emotionally charged atmosphere, Hale said softly to the surgeon, "Doctor, it appears that you know more about anesthesia than I, so I suggest that we change places." The storm clouds parted instantly. The surgeon recognized Hale's wisdom as the patient's unstable condition was corrected.[19]

Hale started a training program in anesthesia for physicians, and one of the early trainees was Dr. Carl E. Wasmuth. It was Wasmuth who replaced Hale when the latter retired in 1967. Wasmuth was head of the department for only two years before he was elected chairman of the Board of Governors. He was followed by Dr. J. Kenneth Potter. While Potter was chairman, the department was withdrawn from the Division of Surgery and a new Division of Anesthesiology was created.[20] When Potter retired, Dr. John F. Viljoen succeeded him. Viljoen, a first-rate anesthesiologist specializing in the care of patients operated on for heart disease, was unable to manage successfully the many and difficult problems of a new division. When he left in 1976, Potter was called out of retirement to hold the division together until a replacement could be found, and he did a commendable job. A search committee recommended Dr. Azmy R. Boutros to the Board of Governors, and in 1977 Boutros began the long task of building the division.

Boutros had climbed the academic ladder at the University of Iowa where he became Professor of Anesthesiology. Reorganization of the anesthesiology program was given top priority by Boutros, retrieving it from the disarray of the mid-1970s. The breadth and complexity of anesthesiology had increased enormously, and Boutros knew that additional staff members were required for clinical responsibilities and teaching. The staff had totaled 15 members when Boutros was appointed, and the number more than doubled in the next six years. At the same time, the number of resident physicians increased from ten to 40. The program is under the supervision of Dr. Arthur Barnes, director of education for the division. From a one-physician department in 1946 has emerged a 35-physician division in 1984. This has been necessary because of the expansion of the hospital, the growth of surgical specialties, the broadening of responsibilities of anesthesiologists, and advances in technology and pharmacology. The result has been vastly improved care of patients.

Notwithstanding the rapid increase in the number of anesthesiologists, the clinical load could not be carried without nurse anesthetists. In January 1969, two of them (Marietta Portzer and Audrey Spence) started a school for nurse anesthetists. The present director is Eileen Cavanaugh, C.R.N.A. Ten to 12 nurses are enrolled in a two-year program. These students are highly qualified, most of them holding master of science degrees prior to entering the program.

There are now 40 operating rooms in the Cleveland Clinic Hospital. Nine are presently devoted to cardiovascular surgery. The expansion to be completed in 1985 will add more. There is one anesthesiologist for every two rooms, except for the cardiovascular and neurosurgical rooms where an anesthesiologist is present in each room. Nurse anesthetists care for patients under supervision of the anesthesiologist.

When the operations have been completed, the patients are moved to a recovery room or to a surgical intensive care facility. Management of these areas is the responsibility of the Division of Anesthesiology. Common postoperative problems are ventilation of the lungs, proper maintenance of blood pressure, and interaction of various drugs, all of them managed under the supervision of anesthesiologists. Other physicians and surgeons may write orders, but these are countersigned by the anesthesiologist because he or she must be continually aware of the patient's status.

Scheduling operations is a function of the division. Optimal use of personnel and equipment as well as the convenience of the surgeon is important. Some patients may have relatively minor operations and return home the day of operation. The operations must be scheduled so that the surgeon's time is utilized effectively and the patient's time is not wasted. "Ambulatory surgery" will continue to increase because it provides for the efficient use of hospital beds and saves money.

A pain therapy unit is staffed by five anesthesiologists on a rotational basis, assisted by trainees. Eight beds are available for this important work. Members of the Departments of Psychiatry, Neurology, and Neurosurgery are also interested in pain therapy and cooperate with the anesthesiologists.

The Department of Cardiothoracic Anesthesia is the only specific subdivision in the Division of Anesthesiology. Because of the large volume of cardiothoracic operations, there was great interest in the field for many years dating from Viljoen's time in the 1960s and 1970s. A separate department was formed in 1976, and Dr. F. George Estafanous was appointed chairman. He is best known for his description of the complication of hypertension following cardiac surgery. Ten full-time anesthesiologists now constitute the staff. Additionally, there are residents in training for a year following completion of the three-year postgraduate training program in anesthesiology. The total number of personnel working in the department is 63, including individuals often not thought of as involved in the field; 20 respiratory therapists, three chest physiotherapists, three electronic technicians, and one clinical engineer.

The department is primarily responsible for respiratory care postoperatively. It has been possible to decrease significant pulmonary complications from 5 per cent or 6 per cent of cases a decade ago to less than 1 per cent today, even though more patients at higher risk than formerly are undergoing operations. Cardiac complications during and after operation have also been reduced. Interest in cardiothoracic anesthesiology has increased. In 1980, 1000 anesthesiologists from many countries came to Cleveland to attend a conference on problems of cardiac anesthesia. The conference was sponsored by the department.

In the 36 years since the Department of Anesthesiology was created in the Division of Surgery, anesthesiology has expanded in scope tremendously. It is now one of the five divisions of patient care in The Cleveland Clinic Foundation. Its aim is to cooperate with the other four divisions in providing care to patients before, during, and after operation.

Division of Radiology

When the Clinic was opened, radiology had just begun as a specialty.[21] The founders selected Dr. Bernard H. Nichols to be the first head of the Department of Radiology. This choice was a singularly fortunate one, for Nichols was one of the country's pioneers in diagnostic radiology. He practiced medicine first in Youngstown, Ohio, and then moved to the White Hospital (now the Robinson Memorial Hospital) in Ravenna, Ohio. There he met Bunts, Crile, and Lower, who were also on the staff of that hospital and often operated there. Nichols became interested in radiology when a Ravenna manufacturing company began making x-ray machines of the primitive hand-cranked variety and put one of these machines at his disposal.

Nichols entered the Army Medical Corps during World War I and, after completing a course in pathology of bone, served as a radiologist. With this background, Nichols joined the staff as a specialist in radiology in 1921. In the next 15 years he wrote 50 papers on diagnostic radiology, 23 of which concerned the then rapidly developing field of the diagnosis of diseases of the genitourinary tract. Energy, honesty, and an amused affection for people combined to make him a popular member of the staff. He had a goatee that gave him such a distinguished air that he was commonly referred to as the "Duke of Ravenna," the town in which he lived.

In 1922, the Department of Radiology was strengthened by the appointment of Dr. U. V. Portmann as director of radiation therapy and by the purchase of the Cleveland area's first 250,000-volt radiation therapy machine. Tall, massively built, handsome, and somewhat intimidating, Portmann generated confidence. He soon became a national figure in radiotherapy, writing as extensively as Nichols did, chiefly on measurement of radiation dosage and on the treatment of cancers of the thyroid and breast. He wrote a widely accepted textbook on radiotherapy.

A third pioneer in radiology, Dr. Otto Glasser, was a biophysicist, and a member of the Research Division. He was described by a colleague as "a giant radiation physicist." Glasser first formulated the concept of a condenser dosimeter for measuring the amount of radiation delivered by a diagnostic or therapeutic radiation device. This instrument was used for calibrating x-ray equipment, a safety measure for the patient and medical personnel. Previously, radiotherapists estimated the dosage on the basis of reaction of the skin; the amount of radiation required to redden the skin being considered to be an "erythema dose." Glasser's concept was implemented by

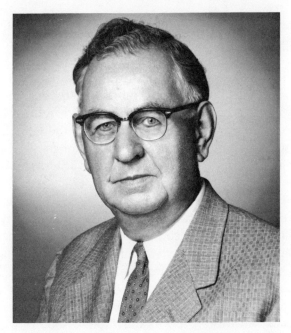

Otto Glasser, Ph.D.   Head, Department of Biophysics, 1923–1964

the Clinic's brilliant engineer, Mr. Valentine Seitz, who constructed a practical unit that was used clinically by Portmann. Thus, the talents of a radiotherapist, a biophysicist, and an engineer were combined to produce one of the fundamental advances in radiology. A prototype of the dosimeter is in the collection of scientific discoveries in the Smithsonian Institution.

Glasser was responsible for control of the radon (radium) seeds used in the treatment of certain types of cancers. He was also a prolific writer of scientific papers and editor of a massive three-volume work entitled *Medical Physics*. Glasser also wrote a definitive biography of the discoverer of x-rays, Wilhelm Conrad Roentgen. Later in his career Glasser's interest turned to radioactive isotopes and again he made important contributions. He was urbane but not pretentious, and he was kindly and considerate to all, relating to those of modest station in life as easily and sincerely as to those of exalted status. His human qualities matched his scientific achievements.

Nichols retired in 1946, and his replacement as head of the

Department of Diagnostic Radiology was a young man, Dr. C. Robert Hughes. Hughes had training in surgery before his interests changed to radiology, and this clinical background combined with his technical knowledge gave him insights valued by internists and surgeons who consulted him frequently about problem patients.

Hughes was a born planner and inventor whose talents were not confined to medicine. During this time, the Clinic was on the threshold of an explosion in growth, and Hughes, working with Dr. Charles L. Hartsock of the Department of Internal Medicine, designed a new facility for the department. Hughes wanted original ideas to supplement his own concepts, so the two planners came up with a unique design that served efficiently for many years with little modification, a great accomplishment in an ever changing field. The Department of Radiology was originally confined to the Clinic building. Only "portable" equipment was used in the hospital, at the bedside, or during operations. A new radiology facility was opened in the hospital in 1947. Surgical operations were becoming more complex, and often it was desirable to obtain intraoperative radiological examinations, and so x-ray facilities were included in many of the operating rooms when the new surgical pavilion was built in 1955.

Dr. Thomas F. Meaney was appointed head of the Division of Radiology in 1966. A young man with innovative ideas, he arrived at his position coincident with tremendous improvements in x-ray technology. He was already recognized widely for his work in angiography. Under Meaney's direction, the Division of Radiology has undergone unparalleled growth. The development of image-amplifying machines led to expansion of the hospital radiologic unit, and in 1974 there was a vast expansion of the department when the new South Clinic building and the new Hospital wing were added. Still further expanded radiologic outpatient facilities will be available in the new Clinic building now under construction (1984), and the department will occupy some space in the new Hospital wing. In 1983 a large gift from Mr. E. T. Meyer, president of The Cleveland Clinic Foundation (1969–1972), made possible the construction of the building that houses the two large nuclear magnetic resonators.

Image-amplifying equipment was the first of a remarkable series of developments that have completely changed the specialty of diagnostic radiology. While cardiologists, led by Sones, were exploit-

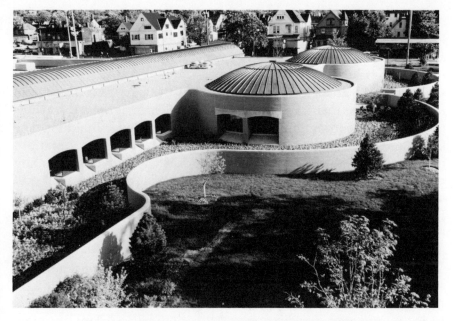

Meyer Medical Magnetic Resonance Center, 1983

ing its value in clinical investigation of the coronary circulation, Clinic radiologists were studying, in other blood vessels, the diseases of the vessels themselves and also the changes in appearance and distribution of the vessels as caused by other diseases, including cancer. Diagnoses could be confirmed that had been impossible previously. In addition, the risk of exposure to radiation was minimized.

In 1972 Meaney visited England to see a scanning device (CAT) that could demonstrate many abnormalities of soft tissue of the brain at no risk to the patient.[22] The fourth such device in the world was installed at the Clinic in January 1974. Although its capabilities extended only to examination of the head, it had a profound effect on the practice of neurology and neurosurgery. Ten months later a body scanner was put in service at the Clinic, greatly increasing the scope of scanning. There is now a fourth generation of scanners, and new uses continue to be found for these machines.

Digital subtraction angiography (DSA) was the next technological pinnacle. The primary advantage over conventional radiography is that an x-ray contrast liquid need not be selectively injected into a particular artery. Rather, dilute concentrations can be used to demonstrate arteries. The injection is usually made in a vein rather than in an artery. The risk of injecting concentrated contrast material into certain arteries, notably those of the brain, is significant. DSA eliminates this risk.[23]

The third great technological feat of the past two decades in radiology is the medical application of nuclear magnetic resonance (NMR). NMR equipment is now in use in the Meyer Building. The Cleveland area is fortunate in having two of the four American manufacturers of this new equipment. NMR will give information not only about anatomical structures but also about normal and abnormal function, including the effect of drugs. A dramatic change in the practice of medicine may well follow the introduction and exploitation of this ingenious device. Its importance may exceed that of the CAT scan.

By the nature of the specialty, much of the radiologist's time is spent looking at images. However, new developments have brought the radiologist back to the patient, especially in the field now referred to as "interventional radiography." It is now possible, for example, to drain the bile ducts by inserting a tube through the skin into the liver, thus avoiding in some cases the necessity for operation. Gallstones may be extracted by an instrument introduced through drainage tubes. Abscesses may be drained by the radiologist. Clots in blood vessels may sometimes be dissolved by dripping a clot solvent around them. Biopsies are obtained using long needles guided by radiologic techniques. Diseases of the lung, kidney, pancreas, and lymph nodes of the abdomen and pelvis may often be identified in this manner, thus avoiding operations.

Contributions of the diagnostic radiologist to medical progress in recent years may be divided conveniently into decades. The 1960s constituted the decade of angiography. The 1970s were characterized by applications of the CAT scanner, the outstanding technological advance of the decade. The beginnings of the 1980s have been marked by the exploitation of DSA and the preparation for another scientific triumph, NMR. It may be predicted that the remainder of the decade will witness a full evaluation of these techniques.

Teaching in the Division of Radiology is an important activity, and 22 physicians are in training in diagnostic radiology. In addition, there is a school for radiologic technicians, a two-year program in conjunction with one of the local universities.

After Portmann's retirement, several therapeutic radiologists headed the department for relatively short periods of time until Dr. A. R. Antunez was appointed department head in 1963. Antunez was a builder, like Meaney. As in the case of diagnostic radiology, radiation physicists and engineers were developing new equipment, and Antunez acquired the latest in equipment, sometimes raising funds to pay for new devices by personally attracting large benefactions from philanthropists and grateful patients.

Today a modern cobalt therapy unit has more than 15 times the power of the original equipment, but a conventional radiation therapy device is still in occasional use. One of the first high voltage linear accelerators for treatment was acquired for the Clinic, and two such units are in use now. Two computers are used in planning proper treatment, and a simulator permits calculation of the maximal delivery of radiation to the desired location. The Lewis Research Laboratories of the National Aeronautics and Space Administration have made available their Cleveland cyclotron for radiation therapy under the direction of our therapists. Its neutron beam has been modified recently to make it the most powerful unit in clinical use. The department consists of five physicians and three physicists.

Some malignancies are best treated by a combination of radiation and chemotherapy, so therapeutic radiologists and oncologists cooperate. Pain caused by cancer often can be controlled by radiation. In addition to clinical research, a specialist in radiation biology is studying the effect of radiation on growth of cells in tissue culture.

The use of radioactive iodine in treating thyroid disease interested Glasser. With Glasser's knowledge and the technical skills of Mr. Barney Tautkins, a hand-constructed rectilinear scanner for the thyroid was constructed. This device worked well and was the beginning of isotope studies at the Cleveland Clinic. A physician was needed to interpret the scans, and the nearest physicians were in the Department of Radiation Therapy, so the isotope studies became a function of that department.

Eventually the gamma camera replaced the slower scanning device, and the development of other isotopes so expanded the vistas of nuclear medicine that a new department was created for such studies, with Dr. Sebastian A. Cook as the first head. Dr. Raymond Go succeeded Cook. The use of the computer has greatly expanded the clinical usefulness of isotope studies in the Department of Nuclear Medicine.

The department has been active in the investigation of the heart by isotope techniques, under the guidance of Dr. W. James MacIntyre, a leader in this field. The motion of the heart creates problems for which special approaches are required. Although a relatively new field, nuclear medicine has greatly contributed to scientific knowledge and to the practice of medicine. Nichols, Portmann, and Glasser would be surprised that from their small beginnings the Division of Radiology has grown to include 21 physicians, four physicists, a computer scientist, a radiobiologist, and three hundred employees who support their work.

Division of Laboratory Medicine

To say that the laboratory is of key importance to the practice of scientific medicine is an understatement. It is better said that the laboratory is at the very center of scientific medicine.[24] The information now provided by monitoring, measuring, imaging, and otherwise analyzing the patient is awesome, and the power of this information to drive the health care system is irresistible. In a nutshell, medical technology lives largely in laboratories, and it is technology that makes possible the diagnosis and rational treatment of disease.

In 1984, the Division of Laboratory Medicine consisted of six departments: Pathology, Immunopathology, Microbiology, Blood Banking, Chemistry, and Laboratory Hematology.[25] There were 43 men and women on the professional staff, either physicians in clinical practice or doctors of philosophy in science (some with both doctorates) who worked with a technical and support staff of 550 persons. All of them occupied a building of 185,000 square feet and generated revenues of $45,400,000. This could surely not have been foreseen in 1921, even by Crile, the most visionary of the founders.

In 1934, Dr. William J. Mayo paid special tribute to surgical pathologists in his address to the first educational seminar on surgical pathology in the United States. In this specialty, the surgeons of the Cleveland Clinic were well-supported by Dr. Allen Graham.

Graham joined the Cleveland Clinic in 1928 as head of the Department of Pathology. He was well known for his abilities as a diagnostician, teacher, and expert in diseases of the thyroid. A trained surgeon himself, he was particularly qualified as a consultant in the operating room.

One has only to review the files he left to see the quality of Graham's service to patients. Several conditions that he carefully segregated are now recognized, having been fully described many years after his work. A special case is that of a woman who had a pulmonary lobectomy done by Dr. Jones about 50 years ago. This case was never fully reported because of the singular structure of the tissue removed. It defies exact classification even now. It is quite probable that no report was published because of Graham's intellectual integrity, such was his concern over not being able to make a diagnosis. He worked alone, even to the point of doing his own microphotography, including development of his films and prints. Autopsy reports were delayed for many months. The workload increased and finally, being unable to delegate work adequately, the burden became so great that Graham left the Foundation in 1943.

During the next few years, the pathology services were ably but remotely supplied by an outstanding pathologist, Dr. Harry Goldblatt of Western Reserve University School of Medicine. Mrs. Ann Haskell, one of the original members of the technical staff of the department, performed many of the routine activities within the department. Although the quality of the reports was excellent, the Clinic surgeons missed the support of a surgical pathologist in the operating room.

Several of the surgical staff had become acquainted with Dr. John Beach Hazard, either in military service during World War II or when Hazard was working in Boston at the Mallory Institute in the Boston City Hospital. Hazard was invited to join the staff, and he did so in 1946. In those days the Department of Pathology was part of the Division of Surgery and was located in an area adjacent to the operating room. Surgeons freely sought consultation either verbally or through the immediate study of frozen specimens. The area occupied by the department, small as it was, was larger than Graham's quarters. Hazard accepted the limitations of available space and set about to organize his department with the enthusiasm and good will that were to characterize his leadership of 24 years.

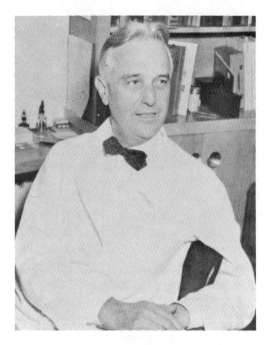

John Beach Hazard, M.D.   Chairman, Division of Laboratory Medicine and
Chief of Pathology, 1946–1970

At first, he was the only physician in the department, but there was a staff of technicians to manage.

Graham had been very uncommunicative, sometimes working for days without speaking to a trainee in his own department. And then there were times when he might open up and startle a listener with his fund of knowledge. Curiously enough, he was an excellent lecturer. In contrast, Hazard was always in an ebullient mood, eager to talk formally or simply to converse in a friendly way on many subjects. His interests spanned a wide field, and so Hazard was approached by colleagues and fellows from many other departments as well as his own trainees. He made pathology come alive. Hazard knew that eventually the clinical laboratories should be combined with his department, but he made no moves to implement this objective that would be self-serving or power-seeking. He had enough to do, carrying the load in surgical and anatomical pathology. For the time being, the clinical laboratories were working productively and efficiently.

The original clinical laboratories were designed by Dr. David Marine. They opened in 1921 under the medical supervision of Dr. Henry J. John, a diabetologist with a keen interest in chemical analysis. Marine never occupied these laboratories.[26] Two technicians, recruited in 1921, worked in the laboratories for more than 40 years. They were Mr. Alfred Reich and Miss Victoria Asadorian. Reich had a degree in agriculture. He served under Marine in World War I and became expert in microbiology and serology. Asadorian was a chief technician in chemistry for 48 years. She retired in 1969.

Henry John left the Foundation in 1933, and for the next decade the clinical laboratories were supervised by Dr. Russell L. Haden, head of the Division of Medicine. Haden was a hematologist and had developed several instruments for the examination of blood. He organized a laboratory for the study of blood diseases. It was located in the Research Building, where Mrs. Irene Sparks supervised the technical work. Haden visited that laboratory every day and carried heavy clinical responsibilities as well. The other clinical laboratories nominally were under Haden's direction, but Asadorian and Reich were actually in charge. In 1944, Dr. Lemuel W. Diggs was appointed head of a new Department of Clinical Pathology in the Division of Medicine. His ideas were incorporated in the design of the modern laboratories within the new Clinic building, and Diggs established the blood bank. Diggs returned to academic life in 1947, and shortly thereafter Dr. John W. King became head of the department. King was well qualified for the post, with a doctorate in bacteriology and a degree in medicine.

Increased specialization, the explosion in basic medical research, and new techniques paved the way for the rapid expansion of laboratory services. In 1940, only 20 laboratory tests were done routinely. During World War II the use of blood, plasma, and plasma products was enormously expanded, and the era of antibiotics began. These two developments profoundly influenced the practice of medicine.

There were other influences. Surgeons required support from the laboratories, and all of the medical specialties required new, rapid, accurate, and often complex tests. King recognized the need for subspecialization within the laboratory itself, and he established a section of bacteriology and serology and a section of biochemistry. Later, an endocrine laboratory was added. King himself headed the section of bacteriology and serology and also the blood bank. Dr. Adrian Hainline became the head of biochemistry, and soon a subsection of microchemistry was formed. The original "special hematology" laboratory established by Haden survived the reorganization of laboratory services, and it, too, expanded the number and range of tests performed.[27]

Expansion of the hospital and its surgical facilities led to increased demand for anatomical and surgical pathologists. Dr. Lawrence J. McCormack joined Hazard in 1951, and Dr. William A. Hawk became the third member of the team five years later. Hazard specialized in diseases of the thyroid, and Hawk focused on gastrointestinal disease. McCormack had wide interests, encompassing diseases of the lung, kidney, bone, and brain as well as the developing field of cytology.

Rapid growth created the possibility of chaos. This was averted when, in 1958, the Foundation created the Division of Pathology. In reorganizing the laboratories, the new division included both the clinical laboratories and anatomic pathology.[28] Hazard became chairman. Specialization continued as Dr. George C. Hoffman was appointed head of the hematology laboratory in 1959. Although morphologic hematology had reached a high degree of excellence, new approaches were developing in bleeding disorders and the hemolytic diseases. Hoffman was noted for maintaining excellent rapport with the clinical hematologists.

Dr. Donald A. Senhauser, later to become chairman of the Department of Pathology at Ohio State University, was named head of microbiology in 1961. Senhauser introduced new techniques in the field of immunopathology.

In 1964, Dr. Sharad D. Deodhar became head of a section of immunopathology. That same year, Dr. Charles E. Willis was appointed head of biochemistry, and three years later Dr. Thomas L. Gavan assumed the role of head of microbiology. Large organizations may at times appear to make unusual choices of executives. On the face of it, Willis was such a choice. Trained as a general surgeon and successfully practicing that specialty, he became interested in clinical chemistry. Though he was proficient, he had started late in his career. He was available for the position of leadership in biochemistry and was chosen. A born gadgeteer, Willis had a talent for working with automatic machinery, getting the most and best

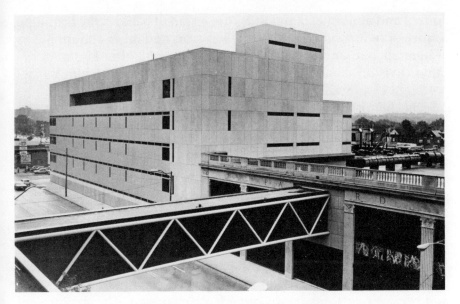

Laboratory Medicine Building, 1980

out of it for the least cost. When Willis retired, Dr. Robert S. Galen became chairman of the Biochemistry Department.

The organization of the division again was revised in 1970 when Hazard retired and McCormack became chairman. The name was changed to the Division of Laboratory Medicine. Hawk replaced McCormack, becoming chairman of Anatomic Pathology. Hoffman, Willis, Gavan, King, and Deodhar remained as department chairmen, as former heads of sections were then to be called. The need for additional space was met first by moving into the old Research Building as a temporary measure. The laboratories were scattered throughout the Foundation's buildings. Plans for a new laboratory medicine building were developed, and the new laboratories were consolidated in this building in 1980. The following year, Dr. William R. Hart became chairman of Anatomic Pathology. In the latter part of 1981, McCormack step ' 'own as chairman by reason of age, and Hoffman was chosen at nis successor.[29]

The hematology laboratory was the domain of Hoffman alone for a long period, but five colleagues joined him, each with specialized interests in diseases of the blood. These interests included intensive study of the structure and the chemical processes within normal and abnormal blood cells, the origin of blood cells, hormone control of red blood cells, sickle cell anemia and other abnormalities of hemoglobin, and abnormal clotting of blood. After Hoffman became division chairman, Dr. Ralph Green succeeded him as department chairman.

Biochemistry, under Galen's direction, has evolved from a single laboratory into five distinct areas. The applied clinical pharmacology laboratory monitors drug levels and toxins, providing also the services of a mass spectrometer. The automated acute care laboratories provide prompt reports of chemical determinations, to guide the proper care of acutely ill patients. The enzyme laboratory analyzes enzymes and isoenzymes in blood serum and other body fluids. Detailed studies of blood fats and proteins are performed in another laboratory. The fifth laboratory is devoted to trace metals. All of these are in addition to the standard biochemical laboratories.

The Microbiology Department replaced the former bacteriology and serology sections, and Gavan is its chairman. The department now has a clinical virology laboratory. The staff of the department has had special interests in antibiotic susceptibility and automation of laboratory services.

Deodhar heads the Department of Immunopathology. This department encompasses the functional study of the immune system of the body, cellular immunity, radioimmunoassay, immune mechanisms in rheumatic diseases, tissue matching for organ transplantation, paternity testing, and cancer immunology with special attention to the control of metastatic disease.

The blood bank prospered under the direction of King when it met the enormous need for blood required by the expansion of cardiac surgery. When King retired in 1981, Dr. Gerald A. Hoeltge became department head. Innovations in conservation of blood by the cardiovascular surgeons have reduced the pressure on the blood bank, even though it is still an active laboratory. New technics in preparation, preservation, and matching of blood and blood products have made these life-saving substances safer than before.

Developments in the five clinical laboratories may appear more dramatic to the casual observer than the developments in anatomic pathology. However, anatomic pathology has progressed in a parallel fashion. From the days when Graham covered all of anatomic pathology, through the period in which Hazard, McCormack, and

Hawk had their own scientific interests, specialization has continued to evolve. All aspects of anatomic pathology are responsibilities of the department, but surgical pathology, cytology, diagnostic electron microscopy, neuropathology, dermatopathology, and cardiovascular pathology are subspecialties within the department. Four members of the staff have divided their special interests among the four areas of gastrointestinal, liver, gynecologic, and orthopedic pathology. Continuity of emphasis on surgical pathology has been maintained by two pathologists, including Hart, formerly professor of pathology at the University of Michigan. New fields of pathology have been opened with the development of immunohistochemistry and electron microscopy. A recent addition is the metabolic bone laboratory.

During his last years as chairman of the division and continuing since, McCormack has been interested in computerization of all laboratory services, assisted by Mr. Walter Hayes. To date, no organization the size of the Foundation has accomplished this successfully. Three of the departments are now operational, and the remainder of the division should be computerized by the end of 1984.

Quality control has been an interest of the Division of Laboratory Medicine for years. The Standards Laboratory of the College of American Pathologists has been located in the Foundation since 1967. The objective is to assure that nationally available products used for laboratory quality control are themselves of high quality.[30]

Residency training, started 40 years ago, now includes 20 trainees in the basic program. Five additional residents are enrolled in special fellowships to gain experience in laboratory subspecialties. A cooperative program with Cleveland State University leads to a Ph.D. degree. A college level training program for medical technicians has been operational for more than 25 years, and graduates of this program are working throughout the United States.

The Division of Laboratory Medicine has been part of the astonishing development of American medical care since World War II. Along with many scientific contributions, the staff has been notable in exploiting new technics of automatic analysis and computerization, at the same time providing support for the other divisions.

EIGHT

"... INVESTIGATION OF THEIR PROBLEMS ..."

Division of Research

Long before the Cleveland Clinic was established, Drs. Crile, Bunts, and Lower supported an active research laboratory with the income from their practices. Crile was the inspiration of the laboratory, and from his investigations came the original thesis that linked the adrenal glands with the adaptation to physiologic stress. Some of the best work ever done in the study of shock came from that laboratory, bringing fame to Crile and, along with so many advances in medicine, underscoring the scientific basis of modern clinical practice.

The founders firmly believed that they could provide the best care to patients by perpetuating an active program of medical research in the new Clinic. They made their intentions plain when, in 1921, they agreed among themselves that no less than one fourth of the net income of the new Foundation would be devoted to research and to giving free care to indigent patients. Later, this percentage was increased substantially, and in 1928 the trustees approved construction of a building to be devoted to medical research.

When the Clinic opened, Dr. Hugo Fricke was in charge of research in biophysics, a field that interested Crile. Differences in electrical charges between the brains and livers of animals and between the nuclei and cytoplasms of individual cells formed the basis of Crile's "bipolar theory of living processes." Fricke, and later Dr. Maria Telkes, measured the thickness of cell membranes and showed their relationship to electrical charges in living cells. These studies were widely recognized as contributions to this complicated field.

As Crile grew older, the biophysics group was replaced by a biochemical team, headed by a young biochemist, Dr. D. Roy McCullagh. McCullagh joined the Clinic in 1930. Encouraged by Lower, McCullagh tried with great persistence to isolate from the testicle a hormone that would inhibit the enlargement of the prostate gland. The quest was tantalizing, but no solid results were ever obtained. McCullagh was a pioneer in the measurement of thyroid function by determining the level of iodine in the blood. He cooperated with his brother, Dr. E. Perry McCullagh, the Clinic's endocrinologist, in the study of pituitary and sex hormones.

The Research Building was designed for the kinds of research that scarcely exist today. By 1945, it had been almost abandoned except for the small laboratories of Dr. Lena A. Lewis, Dr. Otto Glasser, and Dr. Daniel Quiring, and it was in a state of disrepair. During the late 1930s and the early years of World War II, Crile's leadership had waned. He died in 1943. It was possible to keep the laboratories partially serviceable until the end of the war, but the laboratories had neither the resources nor the inspiration that they had when Crile was at the peak of his influence in the Clinic.[1]

Although the founders had passed from the scene by the mid 1940s, their values and their ideals remained. The trustees and the professional staff continued to believe in and to support medical research. But a leader was needed, and it is to the everlasting credit of the trustees that they persuaded Dr. Irvine H. Page in 1945 to become the director of the Research Division of The Cleveland Clinic Foundation.

Page was well known to the Clinic before he came to Cleveland. Dr. Haden, then chief of medicine, had referred a patient, Mr. Charles Bradley, to Page, who was then at Eli Lilly Company and the Indianapolis City Hospital. Bradley belonged to a prominent and public-spirited Cleveland family. He had high blood pressure, and Page was a leader in the scientific work that was unraveling the cause of high blood pressure and thereby establishing its treatment.[2] Bradley's brother, Alva, accompanied Haden on a visit to Indianapolis toward the end of World War II, and Page was invited to come to the Clinic as director of research. When Page accepted, a new era began.

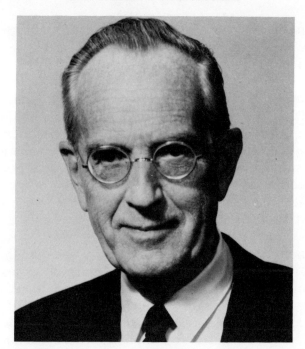

Irvine H. Page, M.D.   Chairman, Research Division, 1945–1966

Page brought two Indianapolis colleagues, Drs. Arthur C. Corcoran and Robert D. Taylor, to the Clinic. They developed a multidisciplinary approach aimed at solving problems in cardiovascular disease. A plan, unique at the time, was devised whereby individuals with specialized training in the basic sciences and in clinical research would work full-time in the cooperative study of diseases of the heart and blood vessels.

Cardiovascular disease, but more specifically, arterial hypertension and atherosclerosis, had been the main interest of Page, Corcoran, and Taylor when they moved from Indianapolis City Hospital in 1945. Page had begun his work in this field in 1931 at the Rockefeller Institute after three years as head of the Chemical Division of the Kaiser Wilhelm Institute, now the Max Planck Institute, in Munich, Germany.[3] Corcoran came to New York from McGill University. Taylor joined Page and Corcoran after they moved to Indianapolis in 1937.

Heart disease had been largely unrecognized until the past few decades. In the 1930s, except for the rheumatic and syphilitic varieties, it received relatively little attention. As recently as the 1930s, high blood pressure was generally considered to be a relatively harmless accompaniment of aging, but by the 1940s the incidence of heart attacks, strokes, and hypertension (and their interrelationships) had become evident to everyone. At that time only a few persons were studying the problem. Page was one of them, working then at the Rockefeller Institute in New York. Corcoran joined him there and studied the renal aspects of hypertension. Sophisticated methods were used for the study of the function of the kidneys in patients with hypertension, and this opened the way to the search for effective antihypertensive drugs and animal models in which new drugs could be tested.

Hypertension was produced in dogs by transplanting the kidney under the skin and then treating it with heavy doses of x-rays. In 1934, Goldblatt, in Cleveland, produced a much more satisfactory model by putting a clamp on the renal artery and partially blocking it. Later Page developed a simple, practical method in which the kidneys were encapsulated in cellophane. This elicited an inelastic hull around the body of the kidney which restricted its normal pulsation and caused severe hypertension.

While still in Indianapolis, Page began to work on the isolation of a substance formed when blood is clotted, a substance known to have a strong action on the circulation. This work was resumed in Cleveland, and with the collaboration of Drs. Arda A. Green and Maurice Rappaport a compound was discovered that proved to be 5-hydroxytryptamine, unknown before. It was called "serotonin." Few biological agents have proved to have so many actions as serotonin. They range from having profound effects within the brain to being the active constituents of certain tumors of the intestine. Many believe serotonin participates in the nervous system as a transmitter of nerve impulses.

A long series of investigations by Page and his associates led to the isolation of a substance that the group named "angiotonin." Concurrently, and unknown to them, another group under Braun-Menéndez in Buenos Aires isolated the same compound. A friendly dialogue between the Cleveland and Buenos Aires laboratories led to an agreement on the name "angiotensin" for this substance. It has formed the basis of thousands of studies, worldwide, and has proved to be a fascinating participant in hypertension as well as the chief regulator of the secretion of a hormone from the adrenal gland. Angiotensin was synthesized both by Dr. F. Merlin Bumpus and colleagues in the Division of Research and by Dr. Robert Schwyzer in Switzerland; thereafter it became widely available for all investigators to study.[4] The achievement was recognized by the sharing of the 1968 Stouffer Prize by Drs. Bumpus, Schwyzer, W. Stanley Peart, and Leonard T. Skeggs.

In the Division of Research, a concerted effort has been made to ensure the cooperation of scientists in several disciplines. Page did not permit departmentalization. Observations of patients (under the care of physicians in the Division of Research), animal experimentation, and work in the chemical laboratory were melded. Page wanted the division as free as possible of barriers to cooperation. He disdained committees, an excessive number of meetings, and other administrative impediments. This freed everyone to participate in the research itself. It took a lot of work to maintain such a seemingly structureless organization, because of the inherent tendency of people to organize, obtain titles, and assume roles.

The research work done today is divided into two categories: (1) program research and (2) project research. Program research is done by the members of the full-time staff of the Division of Research and until 1966 was concerned solely with cardiovascular disease. Project research, in contrast, is conducted by members in the clinical departments. The plan for each project must be submitted in writing and approved by the Research Projects Committee before funds and space are made available. The kind of work undertaken depends on the interest of the investigator and may or may not relate to program research.

Fortunately, the first Research Building was located between the Hospital and the Clinic, thus ensuring frequent and easy contact with the problems of the patients and the clinical staff. In the early years of the division's existence, regular attendance at all the Foundation's medical and social functions was virtually mandatory, but as the Clinic has become larger, there has developed to some degree the usual grouping of persons with similar interests. This phenomenon, which the Clinic's Division of Research is still trying to avoid, occurs to an extreme degree in many universities, with the result that interdepartmental communication breaks down.

For many years, the funds for research came only from the

Foundation. There was active antagonism to accepting support from the government. But in the early 1950s it became necessary to accept federal grants. In 1962, a major program grant was awarded to the Research Division by the Heart Institute of the National Institutes of Health. The funds were not paid to individual investigators, as is customary in many institutions, but to the Foundation. This arrangement tended to eliminate the financial competition among individual investigators. Salaries of most of the staff are paid by the Foundation. This affords security greater than the security of scientists whose salaries are dependent on grants. Grants are used to defray operating expenses. Gifts from individuals and foundations have proved especially helpful.

As Page began to shape the Research Division in his model, he added Dr. Arda Green, who had just crystallized phosphorylase-A while working with Carl F. and Gerty T. Cori in St. Louis; Dr. Georges M.C. Masson from the laboratory of Dr. Hans Selye in Montreal; and Dr. Willem J. Kolff from the Netherlands. Three younger scientists, Drs. Bumpus, Harriet P. Dustan, and James W. McCubbin, came as young associate staff or post-doctoral fellows. They developed their careers at the Clinic.

Kolff had spent the war years in Holland, working on the artificial kidney. Page met him in 1948 and invited him to join the staff in the Division of Research. Fortunately, Kolff was pleased to come to Cleveland. To do research while his country was occupied by the German army obviously took great courage and determination. A stubborn will to accomplish his goals has always characterized Kolff, and he worked against great odds in obtaining funds for his work in those early days. The Cleveland Clinic Foundation was the sole support of the artificial kidney work initially, because very little money was available at that time. An artificial kidney for humans seemed so unlikely that few persons desired to invest in it. Private foundations were the first to see the light, and the National Institutes of Health later became the prime source of funds.

Both Page and Kolff had strong convictions, a trait that would in time lead to conflict. To keep both men highly productive a separation became necessary. Kolff continued his research effort in the Division of Surgery until Page's retirement in 1966.

While Kolff was working in developmental medicine, Page and his group were establishing the Cleveland Clinic Research Division as the mecca for research in high blood pressure. The principle of feedback, now widely applied in engineering and other fields, was early shown to be a part of the intricate mechanisms controlling blood pressure. From many experiments came the general theory of hypertension, called "the mosaic theory." The mosaic theory postulated that hypertension, like atherosclerosis, rarely has one single cause, but rather results from shifts in the equilibria among its many component causes.[5]

One of the unique features of the Division of Research was the development of a plan to integrate care, clinical study, and laboratory investigation. This proved to be a major innovation.[6] It allowed extensive study of the effects of new antihypertensive drugs on a small group of previously studied patients. Drugs such as guanethidine, dihydrodiuril, and hydralazine were launched here and elsewhere, too, as might have been expected in so competitive a field.

Mr. Frederick Olmsted did much in the early development and application of electromagnetic flowmeters. For the first time this allowed measurement of the output of the heart, regional blood pressure, and other facets of the circulation in healthy, unanesthetized animals. This development has done much to advance the understanding of the highly complex mechanisms controlling the flow of blood to each organ.[7]

Blood oxygenation was another development from this same laboratory. It was pursued concurrently with the developing interest in coronary catheterization by Dr. F. Mason Sones, Jr. Conjoint research efforts by Kolff and Sones and by the cardiovascular surgeon Dr. Donald B. Effler advanced the development of modern heart surgery.

A new brain hormone was discovered by Drs. Subha Sen and Bumpus that appears to be another controller of aldosterone secretion by the adrenal gland. As yet, the stimuli for its release are unknown, but recent studies are beginning to unravel its role in some human pathologic conditions.

Research on hardening of the arteries (atherosclerosis), which accounts for the majority of heart attacks and strokes, also has had a long history in the Division of Research. When it became apparent some time ago from the work of others that under certain conditions increased blood fat levels in both animals and man were associated with atherosclerosis, work was directed towards modifying fat levels by changing the diet. Promising results in the laboratory then prompted a pioneering clinical investigation: A small group of co-operative medical students consumed experimental diets developed and supervised by Dr. Helen B. Brown of the Division of Research, and it was found that certain of these diets were effective in decreasing fat levels. The United States Public Health Service became interested in the program and offered substantial financial assistance, eventually assuming the complete cost of a much expanded and expensive program. This dietary project, "The National Diet-Heart Study," showed the feasibility of a much larger long-term program that would involve the cooperative efforts of many institutions. It would ultimately provide the basis for making a recommendation to the American public that a change in its eating habits would help to prevent heart attacks and strokes.

Dr. John R. Shainoff approached the problem of atherosclerosis from another angle, believing that both the initial atherosclerotic lesion of arteries and final closure by blood clots involved fibrinogen, the main substance of fibrin. Little was known about the mechanism of the formation of fibrin or fibrinogen, and this was Shainoff's problem. He discovered that the initial step is the freeing of substances called fibrinopeptides, but as the story unfolds, many new approaches to detection and control of fibrin deposition and clot formation will become available.

The creation of an immunology department was a natural evolution of the Clinic's interest in renal transplantation. Studies on immune rejection naturally relate to cancer and to autoimmune diseases. This department, now the Department of Molecular and Cellular Biology, is evolving a multidisciplinary approach to these diseases and includes staff with training in pharmacology, radiobiology, and molecular biology as well as scientists more oriented toward immunology.

The growing national interest in cardiovascular disease was reflected in the organization some two decades ago of the American Foundation for High Blood Pressure, later to become the Council for High Blood Pressure Research of the American Heart Association. This organization meets in Cleveland annually. The Coronary Club has more recently been organized as a lay-professional organization to give advice and understanding to those who have suffered heart attacks. The annual Stouffer Prize of $50,000, established in 1966 through the foresight and generosity of Mr. Vernon Stouffer and his family, was given to stimulate the highest quality of work in the fields of hypertension and atherosclerosis. The Stouffer Prize has now been replaced by the annual Ciba Award.

The philosophy of the Division of Research from 1945 to 1966 had been steadfastly to maintain the cardiovascular program and add to it approved research projects from any department. After Page retired, additional departments of Immunology (now Molecular and Cellular Biology), Artificial Organs (including Biomechanics), Biostatistics, and Clinical Science were added.[8] This growth necessitated breaking the long tradition to seek no funds from outside the Clinic. The issue of whether or not to do so led to acrimonious debate. But in departing from tradition the new policy has proved to be even more effective than was anticipated.

The environment in which the problems of cardiovascular disease are a continuing challenge is stimulating not only to the investigators but to the clinical staff as well. This environment provides the excitement and the drive for everyone to participate in the understanding of these diseases, statistically among the more prevalent of all illness, and in the care of patients suffering from them. The efforts of the Molecular and Cellular Biology Department are directed largely to problems of cancer and autoimmune diseases. A new department, its full impact is yet to be felt.

Without the strength of basic programs, involving the cooperative efforts of scientists, the Clinic would not have attained its position of national leadership in the medical community. Although project research has been highly creditable, the conclusion to be drawn from a review of the history of the Division of Research is that coordination and cooperation are the key to success. Since Page's retirement in 1966 and the appointment of Bumpus as chairman of the division, applications of these principles have continued to be productive in the development of new lines of thought.

Many physicians and scientists worldwide who are doing important work received their training in the Division of Research. Medical science is an international enterprise. Trainees have come from nearly every country. These international bridges are a stimulus to the professional staff.

In 1974, a new research building was erected. This magnificent

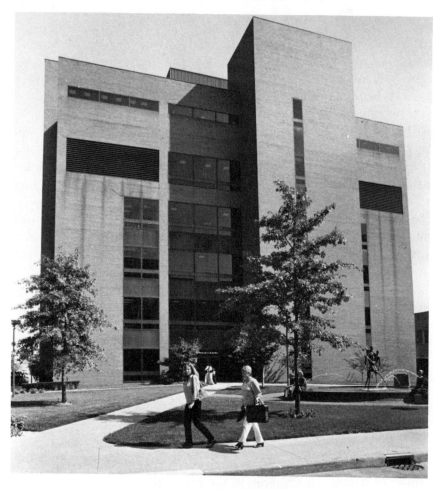

Research Building, 1974

structure, funded by gifts to the Foundation, was filled almost immediately. As with most research facilities, the need for more space is ever present.

NINE

■ ". . . FURTHER EDUCATION OF
THOSE WHO SERVE . . ."

Division of Education

"We hope, too, that as we have after many years been allowed to gather together able associates and assistants to make this work possible, so in time to come, those men, taking the place of their predecessors, will carry on the work to higher and better ends, aiding their fellow practitioners, caring for the sick, educating and training younger men in all the advances in medicine and surgery, and seeking always to attain the highest and noblest aspirations of their profession." These words were spoken by Dr. Frank E. Bunts at the opening of the Clinic in February 1921.

It is not surprising that the founders placed so much emphasis on teaching. All were members of the clinical faculties in one or more of Cleveland's medical schools. From the time the Clinic began, there were graduate fellows-in-training. The first resident in medicine was Dr. Charles L. Hartsock, who served from June 1921 to June 1923.[1] Thereafter, he became a member of the staff, serving with distinction until his death in 1961. The first surgical fellow was Dr. William O. Johnson, and the first resident in surgery when the hospital opened in 1924 was Dr. Nathaniel S. Shofner. Soon after the opening of the Clinic, fellowships in research were also established, and a number of traveling fellowships were awarded, whereby doctors-in-training had the opportunity to visit other clinics and medical centers in this country and abroad.

In the early years of the Clinic, there were no American specialty boards and there was much more flexibility in training programs than there is today. Residents could finish a year or two of training at one hospital and then, hearing of someone at another hospital with whom they would like to work, could apply to train with that person. This apprenticeship system had no formal rules, rotations, or examinations. A young man, well versed in general surgery, for example, could go to a medical center for a few months or a few years and work with a subspecialist until he became thoroughly competent in the subspecialty. Today, the rigid requirements of the various specialty boards make it difficult to transfer from one institution to another.

In the 1920s, interns and residents in most teaching hospitals often were underpaid (if paid at all). The Clinic paid relatively high salaries for that era. Competent technicians were available to do the laboratory studies that occupied so much of the time of those in training elsewhere. There was, therefore, no shortage of applications for the limited number of fellowships offered. Fellows and staff benefited from the apprentice-like relationship that existed in those days.[2] Although formal postgraduate courses were not established in the early years, over 12,000 physicians visited the Clinic for various periods of time between 1924 and 1937.

For teaching, lecturing, and the presentation of papers, the staff recognized the need for a medical library, a medical art department, and a photography department. Each of these was established. A great advance in the educational functions occurred in January 1935 when The Frank E. Bunts Educational Institute, named for the founder and endowed by his family and friends, was incorporated. Its faculty was comprised of members of the professional staff of the Clinic.[3]

Until June 1962 all educational activities were conducted by The Frank E. Bunts Educational Institute. Then, because The Cleveland Clinic Foundation had become well known, nationally and internationally, the Faculty Board recommended that the name of The Bunts Institute be changed to The Cleveland Clinic Educational Foundation. By so doing, it was hoped that physicians here and abroad would associate the activities of the Educational Foundation with those of The Cleveland Clinic Foundation.[4]

With the development of the American specialty boards and the increased activity of the Council on Medical Education of the American Medical Association, formal training programs were established so that the candidates could meet the requirements of the examining bodies in the various specialties. The increase in medical knowledge has necessitated a continuing development of and paralleling increase in the Clinic's educational standards.

During the early years, the fellowship program was administered through a Fellowship Committee. The first such committee was organized in 1924, and Dr. Robert S. Dinsmore of the Department of General Surgery served as chairman until 1936. He was succeeded by Dr. Alexander T. Bunts of the Department of Neurosurgery, who held the post with distinction for the succeeding ten years. Bunts (son of the founder) was then succeeded by Dr. William J. Engel of the Department of Urology. Engel's tenure was short-lived, pending the reorganization of the Educational Foundation.

With the continuing expansion of educational activity, it was deemed advisable to have a full-time director of medical education. The first was Dr. Howard Dittrick, a well-known Cleveland physician, who in January 1944 became director of The Frank E. Bunts Educational Institute. For the next five years, he was in charge of the editorial department, the library, postgraduate courses, the preparation of exhibits, and the art and photography departments. He also edited the *Cleveland Clinic Quarterly*, which had been publishing scientific papers by members of the Clinic staff since 1932.[5]

Upon Dittrick's retirement, Dr. Edwin P. Jordan, who was an editor at the American Medical Association, was appointed director of education. He served in this capacity from September 1947 until July 1950 and was succeeded by Dr. Stanley O. Hoerr until April 1952. Dr. Fay A. LeFevre was acting director of education until 1955, when Col. Charles L. Leedham was appointed director of education. Leedham had spent many years in medical education in the armed forces. In 1962, Leedham resigned as director of education. He was succeeded by Dr. Walter J. Zeiter, former executive secretary of the Board of Governors, who held the position until January 1973.

At Zeiter's retirement, Dr. Thomas F. Meaney became the acting director of education until the arrival of Dr. William M. Michener in July 1973. Michener, a former Cleveland Clinic staff member, returned to the Clinic after five years as professor of pediatrics and assistant dean for graduate education at the University of New Mexico School of Medicine.

Within The Frank E. Bunts Educational Institute was established the Faculty Board in January 1956. The basic function of the Faculty

Board was responsibility for the quality of the educational programs and the development of the policies governing these programs. There were nine members: The chairmen of the divisions, the director of research, the chairman of the Board of Governors, the director of education, and two members at large.

The responsibilities and duties of the Faculty Board were to make appointments and promotions within the teaching faculty composed of the Clinic staff members; to determine educational policies and curricula for the conduct of graduate education; to determine the numbers of interns and fellows to be appointed, as well as to establish criteria for selection of candidates; to establish standards for the granting of certificates for academic work performed at the Educational Foundation; and to appoint necessary committees to advise and assist the director of education through the Faculty Board in the discharge of his responsibilities.[6]

As the years passed with ever-increasing activities in education, many members of the Clinic staff hoped that adequate physical facilities could be acquired for graduate, postgraduate, and continuing education. This dream became a reality with a generous gift from the estate of Martha Holden Jennings for construction of the seven-story Education Building and an endowment to help maintain it. The Education Building contains an auditorium, seven seminar rooms, a medical library, editorial and administrative offices, and bedrooms for house staff on call.

Before construction of the Education Building, four or five postgraduate courses were offered annually, each with a maximum capacity of about 125 physicians. When the new building was completed as many as 20 two-day courses were offered. Attendance increased to more than 2,000 physicians a year. The courses have become highly diversified and specialized. They now encompass continuing education in nearly all specialty fields of medicine and in most of the allied health professions. These intramural educational activities are supplemented by an extramural program: members of the Cleveland Clinic staff participate in the educational activities of many midwest hospitals. By the mid-1980s nearly 12,000 physicians and allied health personnel were reached annually by the intramural and extramural programs.

In 1973, clerkships for medical students were offered. Before that time, few medical students had been exposed to the practice

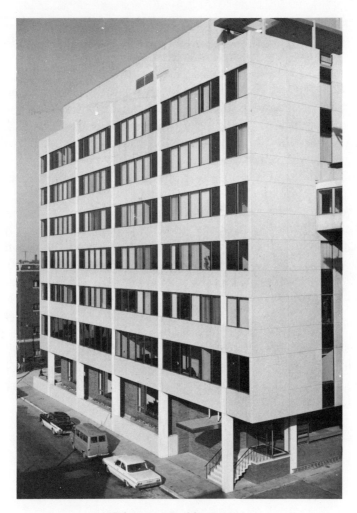

Education Building, 1964

of medicine in the Cleveland Clinic. The clerkships offer medical students the opportunity to participate in integrated group practice as it occurs each day at the Clinic. Now more than 500 medical students from 70 American medical schools participate in this program. A benefit has been the recruitment of many of these medical students into the Clinic's graduate education programs. Approximately 50 per cent of the incoming first-year house staff are former medical student clerks.

The Education Building has long been fully utilized. The auditorium and classrooms are in use from 7 A.M. to 6 P.M. and often longer. The medical library provides bibliographic search services. The Cleveland Health Sciences Library supplements the services of the medical library. The department of scientific publications assists the staff in preparing papers for publication in the *Cleveland Clinic Quarterly* and other scientific periodicals and books. Education programs for the allied health professions have continued to increase. There are now 21 such programs.

The number of doctors-in-training at the Cleveland Clinic now exceeds 500. New medical school graduates (formerly called interns) begin training each year, some remaining as long as seven years. There are 30 training programs for physicians. Each year in June the certificate award ceremony honors residents who have completed their training. Eleven prizes for outstanding performance, excellence in writing, research, and leadership are given. These graduates are practicing throughout the United States and in many other countries.

At the Cleveland Clinic, resident physicians observe private patients, experience the integrated team approach to clinical problems, and are supervised by members of the staff. The number and diversity of clinical problems and the group practice provide an ideal training environment.

■ NOTES

Chapter One

1. An important source for this second edition and for the first edition of *To Act as a Unit* was *George Crile, An Autobiography*, edited with sidelights by Grace Crile (1947). Crile was the author of 650 publications including several books.

2. Crile described the origin of University Hospital (not to be confused with University Hospitals established in 1931) in his autobiography on page 20. "In 1882, three years before I first came to Cleveland, Doctor Weed and the group of associates who had revived Wooster Medical School, having no hospital privileges for their students except the county poorhouse, established University Hospital in two old residences on Brownell Street 'in juxtaposition,' as the catalogue stated in a high-sounding phrase, to Wooster Medical School. This simple hospital had a capacity of perhaps thirty beds."

3. The original Bill of Sale documenting this transaction between Weed's estate and Bunts and Crile, contains archaic language and misspellings which are accurately rendered here in these excerpts. This document is now located in the Archives at the Cleveland Clinic.

4. As Crile prepared to leave for France, Lower drafted a report to be presented to the office staff. The report is less interesting than this draft here reproduced with some minor editing to correct errors. Both drafts are in the Archives of The Cleveland Clinic Foundation.

Partial Report for the Year 1914

In behalf of Drs. Bunts, Crile, and Lower, I want to make

a necessarily incomplete report for the year 1914, incomplete because the year is not entirely ended and because the rush of extra work at this time has made it impossible to get all the necessary data ready. It is only by summing up of the year's work that we can get a keen appreciation of what we have accomplished. I wish you to particularly hear this because of the important part you all have taken in the work.

Your loyalty, zeal, enthusiasm and devotion we have all recognized throughout the year and wish to take this occasion to tell you how keenly we appreciate it and also to get your suggestions, if any, for the coming year.

The great European conflict has had its effect upon practically every line of public endeavor in every country of the globe and will continue to do so, more or less, until the war is ended. This means personal sacrifice, more economy and greater efficiency if we wish to hold our place. Our work is particularly trying because it deals solely with other's afflictions. It means great tact, every consideration for the comfort of our patients, the application of the latest and best scientific and practical means for the alleviation of their ailments; special research and laboratory work, reviewing of the literature, the development of new methods of treatment, and the careful computing of our clinical results, which is a guide as to the value of any method of treatment.

The following statistics show approximately what we have done.

Number of cases seen in 1913—8467

Number of cases seen in 1914—9245

Number of examinations for the Railroad Companies in 1913—3185

Number of examinations for the Railroad Companies in 1914—2378

Number of laboratory tests

Wasserman Reactions 113

Complement Fixation Tests 192

Cystoscopies 105

Ureteral Catheterizations 31

Number of papers read at different meetings—30

Number of articles published in the Medical Journals—30 +

Number of reprints sent out—10,000
Number of books published—2

This office has always felt equal to any emergency or occasion that might arise. During the breaking out of the Spanish-American war, when we were just beginning to feel our way, and trying to take our place in the professional world, Drs. Bunts and Crile gave up their work to serve during the war. It was a big office sacrifice. Upon their return I went into our foreign service for a period of nearly one year. Now the opportunity has again arisen to do our part in the great European war and again we are ready. Dr. Crile with his traditional enthusiasm and resources goes to take charge of a division in the American Ambulance Hospital in Paris. With him goes our great aide-de-camp, Miss Rowland, whose ability and capacity for work we all know. With this important division away, the lesser of us must try all the harder to keep the good work going. It means for the rest of us no let down if the coming year is to make anywhere near as good a showing as this one has.

Chapter Two

1. The charter granted by the State on February 5, 1921, reads as follows:

"THESE ARTICLES OF INCORPORATION OF THE CLEVELAND CLINIC FOUNDATION
"WITNESSETH:

"That we, the undersigned, all of whom are citizens of the State of Ohio, desiring to form a corporation not for profit under the general corporation laws of said State, do hereby certify:

"FIRST: The name of said corporation shall be THE CLEVELAND CLINIC FOUNDATION.

"SECOND: Said corporation and its principal office shall be located at Cleveland, Cuyahoga County, Ohio, and its principal business there transacted.

"THIRD: The purpose for which said corporation is formed is to own and conduct hospitals for sick and disabled persons; and in connection therewith, owning, maintaining, developing and conducting institutions, dispensaries, laboratories, buildings, and equipment for medical, surgical, and hygienic care and treatment of sick and disabled persons, engaging in making scientific diagnoses and clinical studies in, carrying on scientific research in, and conducting public lectures on, the sciences and subjects of medicine, surgery, hygiene, anatomy, and kindred sciences and subjects, accepting, receiving, and acquiring funds, stocks, securities, and property by donations, bequests, devises or otherwise, and using, holding, investing, reinvesting, conveying, exchanging, selling, transferring, leasing, mortgaging, pledging, and disposing of, any and all funds, stocks, securities, and property so received or acquired, charging and receiving compensation for services, care, treatment, and accommodations, for the purpose of maintaining said hospitals, not for profit, and the doing of all acts, exercising all powers and assuming all obligations necessary or incident thereto.

"IN WITNESS WHEREOF, we have hereunto set our hands this 5th day of February 1921

> Frank E. Bunts
> George W. Crile
> William E. Lower
> John Phillips
> Edward C. Daoust"

2. This "landlord-tenant" relationship between the Mayo Foundation and its medical staff was changed in 1970 when, as a result of corporate restructuring, all interests came under the Mayo Foundation.

3. Although Mayo emphasized that the Cleveland Clinic was organized for "better care of the sick, investigation of their problems, and further education of those who serve," he did not phrase it in such a succinct manner. The earliest documented use of this phrase was in 1941 on a plaque dedicated to the founders that was hung at the entrance to Crile's museum.

4. The following is an excerpt from a short history written by Lower in 1928.

"Dr. Crile suggested one day if we could get two houses near together on 93rd Street, not too far from the Clinic, we could fix them up and use (sic) for a temporary hospital. The suggestion was made at noon. At 2 P.M. a patient of Lower's— a real estate agent—came in to see him professionally. After dispensing with the professional visit, Lower incidentally asked if she knew of any property on 93rd Street which might be bought or leased—preferably the latter as we had no money. She said she would find out. She returned in an hour reporting that two maiden ladies down the street had two houses they would be glad to lease as they wanted to go to California to live. Lower gave the agent $100. to go and close the deal. About 5 P.M. of the same day, Dr. Lower asked Dr. Crile about the property he thought he should have. He replied 'Two houses near together on E. 93rd Street.' Lower said, 'I have them!' Crile said, 'The hell you have!' Thus closed the second land deal on 93rd Street and the first step in the formation of a hospital."

5. With the successful completion of the Hospital building in 1924, the Association Building Company had fulfilled its useful life. It had provided the founders with the legal and financial means to construct both the Clinic and Hospital buildings. Since 1921, the Foundation had gradually bought up the stock of the Assocation Building Company. By December 31, 1925, the Foundation owned all common and preferred shares that had at one time represented equity in the old Association Building Company. The founders instructed Daoust to merge all interests into The Cleveland Clinic Foundation. The Association Building Company passed out of existence. Its assets formed the nucleus of an endowment fund that was used to help support research and to finance the charitable services of the Foundation.

6. Lower writes: "The purchase of these. . . houses created a land boom on 93rd Street between Euclid and Carnegie Avenues and no other property was for sale at the prices paid for the parcels already purchased. . . When we decided to build a hospital unit, we had an agent buy land on East 90th Street, ostensibly for garage purposes. We succeeded in getting enough land on East

90th Street for the first unit of the Cleveland Clinic Hospital. From then on trading in land became an interesting game of chess for the Clinic and the property owners on East 93rd Street between Euclid and Carnegie."

7. At a special meeting of the Board of Trustees on Wednesday, December 5, 1928, the following resolution was passed: "Resolved: That we, members of the Board of Trustees of The Cleveland Clinic Foundation, wish to place on record our appreciation of our association with Dr. Frank E. Bunts, who died November 28, 1928.

"Dr. Bunts was one of the four members who laid this Foundation, and who helped to carry it forward to its present condition of power and of influence. The relations of its members to each other have been long and intimate. To one that relation covered more that two score years of precious meanings. With the others, either through professional or professional co-working he held closest relations. To another, Dr. Bunts was a father by marriage.

"In Dr. Bunts were united qualities and elements unto a character of the noblest type. Richly endowed in intellect, he was not less rich in the treasures of the heart. Dr. Bunts had an outspoken religion which was evident in his daily life. His intellectual and emotional nature gave support to a will which was firm, without being unyielding, forceful yet having full respect for others' rights. He graciously gave happiness to others, as well as gratefully received happiness from them. His smile, like his speech, was a benediction. A sympathetic comrade, he shared others' tears, and others' anxieties, and still he was glad and hopeful. Faithful to the immediate duty, his interest was world-wide, covering seas and many lands. Recognized by his professional colleagues as of the highest type of excellence and of service, he was yet humble before his own achievements. Richly blessed in his own home, he helped to construct and reconstruct other homes ravaged by disease. Gratitude for his rare skill, and for the gentleness of his devoted ministries, is felt in thousands of lives restored unto health and usefulness. He loved people and was loved as very few men are by the multitudes.

"His thoughtful judgment and rare kindliness was always

evident at Board meetings and his gracious manner will ever be remembered.

"If, however, we would see his monument, we ask ourselves to look about. Seeking for evidence of the beauty of his character, of the happiness which he gave like sunshine, or of the usefulness of his service, we turn instinctively to our own grateful, loving and never-forgetting hearts." (Punctuation in the foregoing quotation has been edited.)

Chapter Three

1. Dr. E. Perry McCullagh has left the following account:

"It was customary in those days for one of the Staff or a Fellow to accompany the patient to another department. I had gone to the front of the fourth floor with a lady and had introduced her to Dr. Ruedemann. As I approached the balustrade, I heard a rumbling explosion and saw a high mushroom of dense rust-colored, smoke-like gas arise from the center ventilator. I thought at first of bromine. It was clear to me that the masonry building could not burn and that the staff should help the people out and avoid panic.

"The ventilating system connected the basement with all the rooms individually, so that within a minute or so they were filled with the poisonous smoke. The elevator near the front stair was stopped when someone in the power house turned off the electricity and those in the crowded elevator died. The front stairway was crowded with frightened, choking people beginning to panic. Those near the bottom were shouting, 'Go back, you can't get out here—there's fire down here.' There were flames across the front doorway where the partially oxidized fumes met the oxygen of the open air. Most and perhaps all of the people who remained in the stairway died there. A few escaped through the skylight to die later, as did the neurosurgeon, Dr. C. E. Locke, Jr.

"I left the stairway and went into the thick gas on the fourth floor. Those who reached an open window on the west were pretty well off because the breeze was from that direction. I stumbled against a door on the east corridor, and Dr. Edward Sherrer, who was then a young staff member, pulled me in and helped me to hang my head out of the window, which did little good as the fumes were mushrooming out the window. With the help of firemen we were able to get down one of the first ladders to be put up.

"After helping with what emergency care could be given in our own hospital, we searched for our friends, some of whom were alive and many dead at Mt. Sinai Hospital. Many were located at the County Morgue; others were visited at their homes. Dr. Sherrer and I were admitted to the Cleveland Clinic Hospital late that evening with shortness of breath, very rapid respirations and cyanosis. After a few days in oxygen tents, we were discharged, only to be readmitted about ten days after the disaster, and were in oxygen tents again for most of six weeks. This relapse was the result of interstitial edema of the lungs which occurred late in all of those who were badly gassed but survived the first few days.

"Among many of us who were most severely ill, courage and calmness seemed to play an important role in recovery. The lack of oxygen caused loss of judgment and encouraged restless activity, so that those who fought against instructions and the use of oxygen died. The courage and complete disregard of fear in the case of my roommate, Dr. Conrad C. Gilkison, was amazing. We both believed we were dying because everyone up to that time who had developed cyanotic nail beds had died, and we could see our blue nails plainly enough. At 1:00 or 2:00 A.M., both of us unable to sleep, Gilk said 'Perry, if you're here in the morning and I'm not, get old Bennett to take me to the ball game.' Mr. Bennett was the undertaker at the corner of East 90th and Euclid Avenue, a block from where we lay.

"Dr. Sherrer, Dr. Gilkison and I were finally able to return to work about November 15. Recovery of pulmonary function was complete."

2. The sentiment of a Cleveland physician, Dr. Frank A. Rice, who was one of the many local doctors who helped in the efforts to save victims on the day of the disaster, is well expressed in the following letter addressed to Dr. Lower:

May 18, 1929

My dear Doctor Lower:

Our hearts are wrung and we are bowed in sorrow over the loss of your associates, whom we have all learned to love and respect. We feel, too keenly, the pain it has caused you and those of your group who were spared, but we are justly proud of your undaunted spirit to carry on, and out of the ashes of yesterday to erect an institution, bound by traditions, to be a worthy monument to lives and ambitions of its sturdy founders.

I cannot let the opportunity pass without a word of praise and admiration for your nursing staff. I arrived at your hospital as the first of the injured were brot in. Thru out the day, and into the night, I have never seen, not even in 17 consecutive days in the Argonne, such perfect organization. With death increasing horror at every turn, your nursing staff functioned with alacrity, coolness and decision which marked them as masters of their art—truly a remarkable tribute to their institution and your years of instruction.

Yours most sincerely,
Frank A. Rice

Another letter, this one to Dr. Crile, was from Dr. Emory A. Codman of Boston, excerpts of which follow:

I am writing to ask a question.

I always think of you as an eagle able to look directly into the sun, looking down, perhaps, on the rest of us common birds, who are controlled by our sympathies, petty desires, and emotions.

You have climbed the ladder of surgical ambition high into the skies of Fame. You have done more good by your introduction of blood pressure measurements, of transfusion, anoci-association, and gas-oxygen anesthesia than could be counteracted by the death of every patient who entered your clinic in a whole year. In the haste of your upward progress you have known that some wings would break and lives be lost.

Now comes this accident which is not the least your fault and which will do untold good, as every X-ray laboratory in the world will be safer for it.

And now, my question: Since you have known both 'Triumph and Disaster'—did you 'treat those two Impostors just the same'?

To this query Dr. Crile replied:

Referring to our own terrible blow, the only thing that hurts me and that will always be, is the loss of life. I saw nothing in France so terrible. It was a crucible. Almost four hundred people were in the building at the time.

You have always been a close friend. I appreciate you, especially now.

3. A commemorative, *In Memoriam,* was issued by the Board of Trustees in June 1929, eulogizing the victims of the disaster. It reads in part: "The integrity of the Cleveland Clinic Foundation could receive no more severe test than that of the recent disaster. Each member of the medical staff, as well as every employee in every department, has faithfully carried on his or her own task, knowing that the Clinic was not destroyed, but rather that from the ruins will arise an even better institution which will be dedicated as a sacred memorial to the dead."

Chapter Four

1. Crile and Lower did not think that there would be any liability. The storing of the films had been in accordance with the fire laws, and the fumes from films had not been recognized as potentially fatal. In 1928, however, eight persons had died in a similar fire in Albany, New York. Suffocation was believed to have been the cause of several of those fatalities.

2. Crile wrote in 1933, ". . . the one abiding comfort, as I looked at our beautiful cathedral for service, was that during the years that I had needed least and could give most I had been able to earn in such excess of my salary that we had been able to accomplish that of which we had dreamed."

3. Crile's research into the energy systems of animals was supported in part by an endowment received from Sarah Tod McBride. In 1941, the Museum of Intelligence, Power and Personality, was built adjacent to the old Clinic building, to exhibit the specimens that Crile had collected. Dr. Alexander T. Bunts wrote in 1965, "Many parties of school children visited the museum and were fascinated by the mounted specimens of lion, alligator, elephant, gazelles, giraffe, shark, porpoise, manatee,

zebra, and many other interesting creatures. Models of the hearts of race horses and whales, fashioned of paraffin or plaster, and wax models of the sympathetic nervous systems, brains, thyroids, and adrenal glands attracted the interest of the curious and challenged the logical thinking of visiting scientists and physicians. . . . Those of us who were working at the clinic in those days were never surprised to encounter a dead lion or alligator in the freight elevator of the Research building or occasionally even a live one, as well as a battery of vats filled with viscera of various animals. In the study of this material, emphasis was placed on the relative weight of thyroid, adrenals, liver, and brain, and the complexity of the autonomic nervous systems."

Mr. Walter Halle, later to become one of the Clinic's trustees, recalled the following episode:

"I got a call from Doctor Crile one day asking if I would come down to the Clinic and serve in some sort of protective capacity, armed with my Mauser 3006, while they were attempting to uncrate a lion sent to him from the Toledo Zoo. The lion was brought up on an elevator in a cage, in a very irritable condition, and moved into the room where he was supposed to be dispatched in some fashion that had not been too thoroughly worked out. After much thrashing around the lion was quieted and someone gave him a shot to put him away peacefully. I hesitate to think what would have happened had the lion broken out of the cage, which he was attempting to do. Fortunately for everyone we did not have to use our firearms because firing a high-powered rifle in a room 14 × 18, with Doctor Crile and three other doctors, would have made it problematical just who would get drilled.

"I can't tell you what an interesting session I had afterwards watching him dissect the lion and listening to his marvelous running-fire commentary about the glands and various parts of the anatomy."

4. Miraculously no one in that accident died. Crile then made the following observation:

"After the experience of everyone in the plane it seems clear to me that the cause of the blackout in aviation must be the failure of the blood to return to the brain and the heart because of the rapid ascent of the plane. Had I been standing on my head or lying flat with feet elevated and head down—the position used in surgical shock when the blood pressure fails, probably I would not have lost consciousness. . . . Were an aviator encased in a rubber suit and the pneumatic pressure established, the suit in itself would prevent the pooling of the blood in the large vessels in the abdomen and extremities and would maintain the conscious state. I believe that an aviator thus equipped would be protected against the failure of the blood to return to the heart and hence would have protection against blackout."

Crile thought of the pneumatic suit that he had developed years before to treat shock. Why not use such a suit to prevent blackouts that occurred when pilots "pulled out" after dive bombing? The suggestion was passed on to appropriate officers in the Army, Navy, and Air Force. Crile at the age of 77 was made an honorary Consultant to the Navy, and in cooperation with engineers of the Goodyear Tire and Rubber Company produced the first G-suit for military use.

5. Henry Sherman married Crile's sister-in-law, Edith McBride. He was a trustee of The Cleveland Clinic Foundation from 1936 to 1956. He is remembered not only for his wise counsel in the affairs of the Foundation but also for his friendly concern for the professional staff, many of whom he knew personally. Sherman's son-in-law is James A. Hughes, chairman of the Board of Trustees since 1969.

Chapter Five

1. Construction of the portable hospital, all of which was shipped from the United States, was a race against time, for the landing on Guadalcanal was being planned and there would have to be a hospital ready to receive the casualties. For three weeks the physicians and corpsmen labored in the mud of a cricket field in the outskirts of Auckland to put the hospital together. Mi-

raculously they succeeded and were ready when the hospital ship *Solace* brought its first load of wounded. Most of them had had excellent attention, and there was little left to do except give them convalescent care. But there was a lot to be learned about tropical diseases. A young Marine, strong and apparently well, fell sick one day and the next day was dead with convulsions and the meningeal manifestations of malaria.

2. After their tour of active duty, the Clinic paid the returning men their full salaries less the amount paid them by the Navy.

3. Lower expressed the feelings of many when he wrote on the occasion of Crile's death, "George Crile had a quest and a vision that he pursued throughout his entire adult life with a devotion amounting almost to mystic fervor. This is the striking thing that distinguished him from other surgeons and that gave special meaning to his life. He was not content to make use of known truths, but was forever searching for the answer to 'What is Life?' This was the stream into which his tremendous energies flowed, and all his activities and observations were purposeful and tributary to this."

4. The two most powerful figures on the Administrative Board in the 1940s were Jones, Chief of Surgery, and Haden, Chief of Medicine. According to Mrs. Janet Winters Getz, who attended some of the meetings of the Administrative Board in a secretarial capacity, it seemed that these two brilliant and attractive men had agreed to disagree. Sometimes their shouting could be heard over the entire floor. Often the fiery Ruedemann would add his bit. He was a particularly colorful and outspoken man, as exemplified by a story that is told about him when he was in medical school. When asked about the blood count of a patient with leukemia, he reported that the white cell count was 500,000. "Did you count them?" his professor asked. "Hell no, I weighed them," said Ruedemann.

5. Few beds were added by the new wing, however, as much of the space was taken up by elevator shafts designed to serve future additions.

6. Mrs. Janet Winters Getz, who at that time served as Dr. Lower's secretary, stated that he refused to allow their representatives on his floor or to permit any of the personnel on his corridor to talk with them. Yet the firm's report, when it finally came, was constructive. Although it was not accepted in full (the staff was opposed to the suggestion that there be a medical director) it paved the way for the development of a committee system. With the death of Lower in June 1948 at the age of 80 years were severed the last personal ties to the origins of the Clinic. The era of the founders had passed, and the Clinic was on its own.

7. On September 19, 1947, the Executive Committee, in cooperation with the Administrative Board, made appointments of professional administrative officers: (1) Thomas E. Jones, chief of staff, surgery; (2) Russell L. Haden, chief of staff, medicine; (3) Irvine H. Page, director of research; and (4) Edwin P. Jordan, director of education. A professional policy committee was organized to "consult with, advise and make recommendations to the Board of Trustees or the Executive Committee on major professional policies regarding the operation and activities of the hospital and the clinical, research and allied departments of the Foundation." The first membership of that committee consisted of Jones, Haden, Ernstene, Gardner, Page and Jordan.

8. Crile, Jr. recalls the trustee involvement in the reorganization of the Clinic in the late 1940s.

9. The trustees became more active than they had been in Clinic affairs with a view to establishing rapport between themselves and the staff. The Executive Committee of the trustees and the Professional Policy Committee held frequent joint meetings. Subcommittees of trustees and staff members considered many of the problems involving property, facilities, research budgets and the hospital. A fundamental of the new plan of organization was that policies were established by committees. For nine years this form of administration continued.

10. The complex relationships among the consumer, provider and payer that now characterize American health care were only

foreshadowed in the 1950s. In earlier times the ethics of the doctor-patient relationship were often cited in sharp criticism of the Clinic by competing or outside doctors.

11. The members of this committee were: Mr. Richard A. Gottron (Chairman), Drs. Robin Anderson, Victor G. deWolfe, C. Robert Hughes, Alfred W. Humphries, Fay A. LeFevre, Ausey H. Robnett, John F. Whitman, Walter J. Zeiter and Mr. Clarence M. Taylor (ex officio).

12. A quotation from the preamble of the report states that "The Cleveland Clinic Foundation is celebrating its 34th Anniversary this year (1954). Under the leadership of its four dynamic founders it pioneered in the practice of group medicine and laid the ground work which has brought it world renown. Many changes have taken place since the Clinic's founding days. Its physical plant has expanded immeasurably and is in the process of further expansion. From the original four men has grown a medical staff approaching 100. Instead of four successful rugged individualists, the staff now consists of 25 times that number, perhaps less successful, perhaps less rugged, but nonetheless individualist. In many organizations faced with the loss of the leaders who were their creators, a time for appraisal comes somewhere around the 30th year of their history. It is desirable to pause then for some serious thought as to whether the institution continues to carry on the ideals which made it great, and if so, whether it is doing only that or is actually continuing to aggressively meet the challenge of the future."

13. The Medical Survey Committee identified administrative and medical practice issues they felt were critical to the continued success of the Clinic's development. The report recommended that

- the government of The Cleveland Clinic Foundation must become more democratic, so that every member of the staff will feel a greater responsibility for the welfare of the institution and have a more definite stake in its future

- the legal status of the Clinic must be clarified

- the Clinic research and educational programs must be reevaluated and strengthened where possible, since the professional eminence of the institution depends in large measure upon their accomplishments

- the financial well-being of the professional staff must be evaluated to determine whether or not it is adequate

- the Clinic should evaluate the medical needs of the area served, and modify its services to fit these needs

- the Clinic must make a vigorous effort to improve its relations with patients and with physicians both in local and outlying areas

- the Clinic must increase its efforts to keep the public informed about its services, facilities, and achievements

- patient care in the Cleveland Clinic Hospital must be improved.

14. The Board of Trustees in consultation with the Professional Policy Committee recommended that the staff elect members of a Planning Committee, with three members from the Division of Medicine, three from the Division of Surgery, and one from the Division of Research. It was suggested also that members represent varied groups in terms of years of service and include some of the younger men. Those elected were Drs. A. Carlton Ernstene, Fay A. LeFevre, Robert D. Mercer, Robin Anderson, John B. Hazard, W. James Gardner and A. C. Corcoran, with five alternates, namely: Drs. Harold R. Rossmiller, Arthur L. Scherbel, William J. Engel, Stanley O. Hoerr and Irvine H. Page. The trustee membership consisted of the Executive Committee of the Board of Trustees. Donald H. McLean, Jr., an advisor of John D. Rockefeller, III, was appointed to the Board of Trustees and made chairman of the Planning Committee. Richard A. Gottron served as secretary.

15. The plan also proposed formation of committees for research, the hospital, properties, education and planning. The committees would be composed of trustees and members of the professional staff.

16. During the early deliberations of the Planning Committee, it became quite clear that there were certain ancillary professional services that could not be separated from professional responsibility. These areas included the following: central appointment desk, routing desk (including information and patient registration), professional service personnel (including clinic nurses, medical secretaries, and desk receptionists), records and statistics, telephone operators, and patient relations.

     The work of the Planning Committee was greatly facilitated by a study of the structure and operation of the Mayo Clinic, in which a board of governors had been the responsible body of government since 1919. From this study, with due regard for the differences that existed between the two clinics, a plan of organization was developed and adapted to the corporate structure of the Cleveland Clinic.

17. The Board of Governors was given authority to select and appoint new members of the staff, but the setting of the salaries of these and all other members of the staff remained a function of the Compensation Committee of the Board of Trustees. To aid this committee in evaluating the performance of each member of the staff, the Board of Governors was authorized to discuss each member and rate his or her performance, not in respect to the number of patients seen or money earned, but in respect to his scientific and other achievements, so that, in effect, the performance of each staff member would be judged by peers.

18. In the professional area an effort was made to diminish the authority of the chiefs and to encourage individual initiative. Thus the Chiefs of Medicine and Surgery, who theretofore had had absolute authority in their divisions, became chairman respectively of the Medical and the Surgical Committees that were elected annually by the members of their respective divisions. These chairmen were appointed by the Board of Governors for a period of a year, but almost without exception the appointments were renewed annually. Short of illness or mismanagement, the divisional chairmen had what amounted to tenure in their offices. Yet they did not have total control, for they had no authority to act completely independently of their committees. They could be out-voted. Moreover, the actions of the

committees were subject to review by the Board of Governors. This afforded protection to the individual staff member from the capricious or unfair treatment of the chiefs.

19. In 1969 the Division of Research was brought under the control of the Board of Governors.

20. The names of the nominees were sent to the staff for approval and thus was created the first Board of Governors composed of Drs. Fay A. LeFevre (chairman), William J. Engel (vice chairman), George Crile, Jr., A. Carlton Ernstene, W. James Gardner, E. Perry McCullagh and Irvine H. Page. Dr. Walter J. Zeiter was elected executive secretary, and Mrs. Janet Winters Getz was elected recording secretary. The first meeting was held on Thursday, December 8, 1955, at 12:15 p.m. in the Board Room of the Main Clinic Building. In attendance by invitation were Richard A. Gottron, business manager of the Foundation, and James G. Harding, director of the Hospital. Thus began a new era.

Chapter Six

1. Gottron was ill at this time, seriously suffering from an unrecognized depression.

2. Gottron, when replaced by Nichols, was given the job of president of the Motor Center Company, a subsidiary operation of the Clinic. Not long thereafter he took his own life.

3. There was no other physician administrator. Wasmuth recalled that he relied heavily on Messrs. James E. Lees, Robert J. Fischer, and Paul E. Widman when he became chairman. However, Wasmuth reserved ultimate administrative control for himself. Lees functioned as an executive assistant, Widman as director of operations, and Fischer as treasurer.

4. The Cleveland Clinic Foundation gave one million dollars in aid and assistance to the Forest City Hospital, a hospital struggling

to keep operational as a provider of care to many of the urban poor. This hospital later closed its doors. The Collinwood Eldercare Center was partly supported and staffed by the Clinic, and in cooperation with the Cuyahoga County Hospital System the Clinic helped to establish and maintain the Kenneth Clement Family Care Center. A neighborhood revitalization effort, the Fairfax Foundation, received both financial aid and operational assistance from the Clinic.

5. A conflict with the local health planning agency, then called the Metropolitan Health Planning Corporation, was over the issue of the Foundation's right to add 173 hospital beds in the new South Hospital. Although the Clinic prevailed, it was an unpleasant experience and attracted unfavorable public notice.

6. The key administrative team that kept the Clinic running smoothly and tended to the details in those early years of the Wasmuth era consisted of John A. Auble, general counsel, and Gerald E. Wolf, controller, as well as Fischer, Lees, and Widman. Neither Wasmuth nor any other chairman could have functioned without them.

7. The distinction between policy-making and the implementation of policy has been an important development. It has happened because there has been a conscious effort by institutional leaders to define carefully what the responsibilities are for all groups and individuals and to place accountability appropriately. This has not been easy to do. Doctors are trained in their formative years not only to decide for themselves what is the right thing to do (policy) but to involve themselves in doing it (operations). Training programs have been established for the Clinic doctors, not to undo their dynamic approach to patient care but rather to add to their abilities in managerial skills. These programs have been very popular.

8. The Compensation Committee of the Board of Trustees is regularly informed about the Annual Professional Review of the staff. Since 1975, trustees have been advised by the consulting firm of Towers, Perrin, Forster and Crosby, specialists in exec-

utive compensation programs. The reviews and the consultants' reports have been key elements in the salary program for the staff and key administrative personnel. Better organized and administered than in the past, the review of salaries and benefits is one of the most important activities of the trustees.

9. The document that resulted from this study was called the Master Plan. Completed in 1980, it defined the projected expansion and the facilities needed. The Metropolitan Health Planning Corporation approved the construction of a hospital addition of 450 new and replacement beds.

10. In 1979, Congress passed legislation (P.L. 96-79) referred to as the National Health Planning and Resources Development Act, wherein the Cleveland Clinic could be identified as a National Health Resource.

11. The mission statement reads: "The mission of The Cleveland Clinic Foundation is to provide specialized patient care of high quality in a setting of education and research and to continue these activities as an independent, self-supporting institution."

Chapter Seven

Division of Medicine

1. McCullagh remembers that "In spite of (Phillips's) appearance of calmness, there was considerable tension. For example, when he was dictating, no one dared to interrupt. At the end of a busy day his friendliness shone through clearly. He liked very often to sit down in a corner somewhere with his younger staff and fellows. For the first time in the day, so far as I know, he would light a cigarette. For half an hour he would relax and chat of matters of current interest or medical topics. He spent almost all his weekends visiting patients at their homes or in consultation in Cleveland or in neighboring cities."

2. Dr. John P. Tucker was Phillips's first appointee to the medical department. Drs. Oliver P. Kimball, Harry M. Andison, John P. Anderson, Charles L. Hartsock, Robert H. McDonald, and Edward L. Sherrer soon thereafter joined the Division of Medicine.

3. The medical fellow (resident physician) coming to the Haden service did so with apprehension because the "chief" demanded high performance. This challenge brought out the best in the young physician, sometimes surprising himself. Small mistakes Haden never seemed to forget and frequently reminded the offender of them a year or more later, but gross errors might not be mentioned subsequently because he knew how miserable the trainee felt and the lesson had been learned. He never complimented the fellow or chief resident for a job well done, but the young physician knew that Haden was proud of him by the twinkle in his eye and a slight smile. Occasionally he would give an old but valued medical book to a favorite, who otherwise was treated no differently from his peers. Whether in Cleveland or at a medical meeting elsewhere he never failed to introduce his "boys" to his distinguished medical friends.

4. For the alert, serious student Ernstene was a model of uncluttered, perfectly logical judgment. If one listened carefully and attempted to imitate his approach, one learned. He was not a good teacher in the traditional sense. His lectures were excellent because of superb organization and precise delivery. He had a large practice and other responsibilities that crowded out first his investigative interests and then later his writing.

5. These departments were Internal Medicine (1949), Pediatrics (1951), Peripheral Vascular Disease (1952), Rheumatic Disease (1952), Hematology (1953), Hypertension (1959), and Pediatric Cardiology (1960). By 1984, there were some modifications of these names. Pediatrics had become Pediatric and Adolescent Medicine, Hematology had become Hematology and Medical Oncology, Hypertension had become Hypertension and Nephrology, and Rheumatic Disease had become Rheumatic and Immunologic Disease.

6. The Board of Governors decided that something had to be done

to remedy the bad feelings among Kolff, Effler, and Sones, so it formed a committee. The chairman was Dr. William L. Proudfit, a cardiologist on speaking terms with each of the dissident colleagues. The four men met daily at 8 A.M., and Kolff, Effler, and Sones often would talk to each other only through the chairman. Equanimity did not reign, but at least decisions could be made. High risk patients were being operated on, and some patients who had been expected to live had died. At one point, Effler decided to stop operating. Dr. John W. Kirklin, then at the Mayo Clinic, said there was nothing wrong with the approach or the selection of patients and that operations should be resumed. His judgment was correct, and with improved results, bad tempers eased. The morning meetings were discontinued, never to be resumed.

7. Surgical treatment for one type of congenital heart disease proved successful in 1938 and for a common valvular defect (mitral stenosis) a decade later. Open-heart surgery was a development of the 1950s. Kolff had been interested in an artificial heart for some years, and when some means of maintaining blood pressure with an external pump was necessary, it was Kolff who provided the expertise and the equipment. He showed that the heart could be stopped by perfusion with a potassium solution and its action restored by washing out the potassium. Effler was an experienced cardiac surgeon and Sones was an outstanding pediatric cardiologist. These three physicians were positive, strong willed men who did not always hold mutually compatible opinions. In all new fields, errors are made, and open-heart surgery was no exception. Undesired results bred distrust among the three colleagues to the point that for a period of time unemotional communication was not possible.

8. The South Clinic building was planned and built for the two cardiology departments and the Department of Thoracic and Cardiovascular Surgery. Completed in 1974, this addition facilitated the smooth flow of constantly increasing numbers of patients. Five cardiac laboratories were on the second floor of the hospital immediately adjacent to the South Clinic building. The coronary care unit, the cardiac surgery intensive care unit, the cardiac anesthesia department, and the cardiothoracic operating

rooms were convenient to each other and close to the cardiac laboratory. The electrocardiographic, echocardiographic, and stress testing laboratories were adjacent to the offices of the clinical cardiologists on the first floor of the south building. Later were added a pacemaker section and a radioisotope testing area.

9. Growth in cardiology has continued with work being done in pediatric cardiology and in electrical studies of cardiac impulse formation and transmission. Digital subtraction angiography has been added to the other laboratory methods. Clinical research interests have been in studies of the natural history of medically and surgically treated patients with coronary disease, arteriographic documentation of progressive narrowing of coronary arteries, technics of diagnosis and treatment of spasm of the coronary arteries, two-dimensional echocardiographic applications, isotope documentation of contraction of the heart, digital subtraction radiographic technics, and drug testing for control of irregularity of the heart. An information registry is maintained for all patients who have catheterization of the heart or a cardiac operation.

10. The discovery a few years earlier at the Mayo Clinic that cortisone was beneficial in the treatment of rheumatoid arthritis was the basis of new optimism and interest in this and related disorders. Scherbel was trained at the Mayo Clinic.

11. The clinical use of dimethylsulfoxide (DMSO) in the Department of Rheumatic Disease placed the Clinic in the middle of a large controversy. An effective treatment, DMSO figured prominently in the regulatory policies of the Food and Drug Administration. Standards of safety and efficacy and policy regarding the introduction of new drugs were brought sharply to national attention by the birth defects caused by thalidomide.

12. Goiter was endemic in many parts of the United States, and it was not until the importance of iodine was demonstrated that it virtually vanished. Dr. Plummer, of the Mayo Clinic (1920), was a discoverer of iodine's role. Drs. Banting and Best, of Toronto (1922), discovered insulin.

Division of Surgery

13. Although operating in the patient's own room was first devised as a means of avoiding thyroid crisis in patients with hyperthyroidism, it was soon used for all types of goiter, for there were far too few operating rooms for the number of patients needing operations. Crile performed the average thyroidectomy in about ten minutes, then left the resident physician to stop the bleeding and close the wound. This often took half an hour, with the result that it would have been impossible to perform 20 to 30 thyroid operations in a morning if all of them had to be done in the four regular operating rooms.

14. The surgical suite that Dinsmore planned remains a model of simplicity and efficiency and a lasting monument to his foresight and good sense. At the time of Dinsmore's death in September 1957, Crile, Jr. wrote:

> On the ocean it is easy to see the crest of a wave or to feel the surge of a ground swell, but the full flood of a tide may be almost imperceptible even to those who are borne upward on it. Greatness in a man may be, like a tide, so vast and so gentle as to be difficult to perceive.
>
> In the profession of surgery there are technical proficiencies which like waves, crest and fall in the plain view of all. There are ideational advances that, like ground wells, rise higher than the waves and have effects that are more prolonged. But the greatest and most lasting contributions come from those who have the human qualities that mold, lead, and inspire effective teams.
>
> The surgical tradition that Dr. Dinsmore built is a flowing tide that will rise even higher than he dreamed. Perhaps the greatest tribute to his genius is that when he retired he left no technical gap to fill.
>
> Dr. Dinsmore realized that surgery is like a rainbow; it disappears when the sun changes its slant. He knew also that when the rainbow disappears it really is still there and that all you have to do to see it again is to keep moving in the right direction. It was this principle of constant change, of specialization and growth that was the dominant policy of his direction.

15. Chiefs, heads, chairmen, and directors are difficult terms to follow in the history of the Clinic. These terms were official for

differing periods of time and in respect to different positions. By the 1970s, the term "head" was officially abolished to describe the leaders of divisions and departments. These leaders would henceforth be known as "chairmen." The term "head" remains to identify the leader of a section within a department. In casual speech, one can be referred to as the "head" of anything, even though the official title may be something different.

The Clinic has always used the term "division" to describe the larger of the two entities, divisions and departments. The reverse is generally found in other multispecialty medical clinics and virtually all universities. In the Clinic in 1984 there were 28 departments within the two large divisions of Medicine and Surgery. In the early 1970s, there was some talk of switching the terms, but sentiment on the part of the department chairmen and a long tradition of usage made any change unacceptable. The term "division," to describe the larger entity, is common in industry and large organizations other than universities.

16. Ruedemann and Jones were antagonists (note 3, Chapter Five). The reason Ruedemann left Cleveland was due in part to the confrontations with Jones who, of the two, was politically stronger.

17. Effler was approaching his 60th birthday, a time when, as Clinic policy had determined, department chairmen must step down. He left the Clinic to continue his career at St. Joseph's Hospital in Syracuse, New York, where the Clinic's policy of mandatory retirement at age 65 would not reach him.

Division of Anesthesiology

18. A major improvement in the technic of administering anesthesia was the development of endotracheal intubation. The use of curare and the later development of similar drugs permitted controlled breathing via these tubes in patients who were intentionally paralyzed. Intravenous injection of barbiturate drugs to render patients insensitive to pain was a step in what became an important clinical technic employing many other drugs. The

anesthesiologist had to be well versed in physiology and pharmacology.

19. With new technics in anesthesia, new and extensive operations, no physicians to assist him, and a large surgical schedule, Hale faced an almost impossible task in 1946. Gradually conditions improved as result of his efforts, and anesthesia became more efficient and safer than ever before.

20. The Department of Anesthesiology became independent of the surgeons in 1970, but surgeons and anesthesiologists are inextricably intertwined professionally and so their administrative independence was scarcely an escape! The new division was a first step in what has been a long and sometimes painful process of clarification of responsibilities and appropriate behavior in the operating room. The anecdote of Hale's rejoinder to a surgeon's ill-tempered complaint is a good example of what can happen in the stressful atmosphere of an operating room.

Division of Radiology

21. At least one of the founders of the Cleveland Clinic had reason to believe that good diagnostic radiology was essential to the practice of medicine. In 1902, when Crile was still operating at St. Alexis Hospital, one of the trustees of the hospital woke up at midnight, choking, and felt certain that he had swallowed his lower denture. For an hour and a half he clawed at his throat, mistaking the hyoid bone for the missing teeth. He succeeded in so traumatizing the throat that he could no longer swallow, even his saliva. A roentgenogram was made (this was only seven years after Roentgen's discovery of the x-ray) and the film showed some calcifications in the aortic arch which were interpreted as being the missing teeth. The patient was now in serious condition as a result of his own and his physician's attempt to locate and remove the teeth. Finally Dr. Crile was called and was prevailed upon to operate.

   Shortly after the operation the teeth were found in an obscure corner of the patient's room. The next day the patient died and the story hit the headlines throughout the country: "Death Due to Operation. Patient Who Didn't Swallow His Teeth is Dead." Dr. Crile in his autobiography summarized the diagnostic problem as follows:

The positive statement of an intelligent man, a benefactor of the hospital, one whom we had known for a long period, that he had not only swallowed his teeth but that he had touched them a number of times with his fingers and at one time had almost succeeded in removing them; the firm belief of his doctor, a physician of wide experience, that the teeth were still in the throat; the statements of the family that the teeth were not in the room, and their reiterant belief that the teeth had been swallowed, the rapid increase and gravity of the symptoms of the patient during the first day, seemingly out of proportion to the exploratory traumatism; and lastly the positive x-ray diagnosis, overruled our negative findings at the exploration. In consultation the various doctors who had been interested in the case agreed that an operation was indicated.

22. Computerized axial tomography, or CAT, is dependent on the technology of nearly instantaneous processing of enormous amounts of data. Relatively low doses of radiation which pass through sections of the body provide data for imaging.

23. The majority of DSA studies done at present involve demonstration of the arteries to the brain or of the brain, but the arteries of the kidneys and other major vessels are frequently examined. The heart may be investigated by special technics (required because of its motion).

Division of Laboratory Medicine

24. In the context of this assertion, a laboratory is any place where patients, or where elements from patients, are examined and compared with the normal, or are studied in search of clues or new data. Radiology laboratories, clinical laboratories and pathology laboratories with their many technologies are *all* at the

center of modern medicine. This section of the history focuses only on the Division of Laboratory Medicine (of which radiology is not a part), and the role of radiology as a laboratory specialty is not thereby intended to be diminished in any way.

25. Most medical centers, even large ones, do not have as large a laboratory as does the Cleveland Clinic. The more specialized the institution, the more demands are placed upon the laboratories. The annual rate of growth of laboratory studies has been about 15 per cent for several years, seriously adding to the cost of health care not only in Cleveland but nationwide.

26. Marine and Graham served together as resident pathologists at Lakeside Hospital and held concurrent appointments at the Western Reserve University School of Medicine. Although Marine designed the laboratories for the Clinic, most probably at Crile's request, he left the Cleveland area in 1920 to become Director of Pathology at Montefiore Hospital in New York.

27. When Haden left the Clinic in 1949, the unusual arrangement of supervision of the laboratory by hematologists rather than clinical pathologists was preserved. Dr. John D. Battle directed the laboratory, and in 1953 Dr. James S. Hewlett shared these duties. Dr. George C. Hoffman joined the Clinic in 1959 as head of the hematology laboratory.

28. The Divisions of Medicine and Surgery each had a stake in "their laboratories." The reorganization meant that each had to give up something that for years had meant control and revenues. Because of the Clinic's tradition of pooled income, the more significant issue was one of control. This same issue was to be faced when the surgeons "gave up" the control they held over the anesthesiologists upon the establishment of the Division of Anesthesiology (1970).

29. The choice of a clinical pathologist to be chairman would have been considered heretical in the past. Anatomical pathologists dominated the leadership of the laboratories in American hospitals, and as a general rule still wield the most power.

30. Quality has a very high cost. It is not generally appreciated that in a laboratory of the highest standards as much as 40 per cent of all budgeted expenses are directed to meeting the costs of maintaining accuracy!

Chapter Eight

1. Buildings and equipment have been steadily improved but continue to become rapidly outdated because of the speed of current changes in research methods. However, the experience of the division has shown that fine research can be done even without the luxuries which are considered necessities for most modern buildings.

2. Results of clinical studies suggested that there were many causes of hypertension. Chemical substances in the brain, blood, and urine were studied in an extract of kidney first prepared by Tigerstedt and Bergman in Sweden (1898). This substance they called "renin." Page had attempted to purify and isolate the active principle from the renal extracts (1931). He continued the work on purification in collaboration with Drs. Helmer and Kenneth Kohlstaedt in Indianapolis (1937). It was shown that renin was an enzyme unable to raise blood pressure by itself. It could do so only after acting upon blood plasma.

3. The Kaiser Wilhelm Institute led the world in the early researches into the chemistry of the brain.

4. A number of the research staff have spent much of their careers becoming world experts in renal-adrenal blood pressure control mechanisms. Bumpus theorized as early as 1956 that a blockade of this system would lower pressure. He demonstrated this by developing the first molecular antagonists to angiotensin. This encouraged pharmaceutical companies to develop converting enzyme inhibitors that are now evolving into useful drugs for lowering blood pressure.

5. Dr. Carlos Ferrario joined Page and McCubbin in 1966. Page retired not long thereafter, but the investigations they began culminated in a brilliant series of cooperative experiments involving a former associate, Dr. C. J. Dickinson of London. Ferrario, Dickinson, and McCubbin proved that the brain was a regulator of blood pressure. Later, Ferrario and McCubbin showed where and how angiotensin enters the brain. The blood vessels, heart, sympathetic nervous system, brain, pituitary gland, and kidneys are among the complex of contributors to what is called high blood pressure or hypertension. The interrelationships are now being understood.

6. One of the main contributions, with the initial help of a urologist, Dr. Eugene F. Poutasse, was the development of the field of renal hypertension due to obstruction of the renal arteries. Surgical removal of the obstruction often effected a cure. Dr. Thomas F. Meaney, a radiologist, provided the angiograms that were critical to the visualization and evaluation of these obstructions.

7. The study of flow and pressure within the cardiovascular system (hemodynamics) has been one of the cornerstones in hypertension research. High blood pressure is a hemodynamic abnormality, and most of our understanding of its problems requires accurate evaluation of the hemodynamic patterns associated with different types of rise in arterial pressure. Hemodynamic studies have been pursued in experimental animal models and in man, allowing some understanding of the role of the heart in hypertension.

   The "hypertensive heart" has always been a problem in uncontrolled hypertension. Cardiac enlargement occurs. Drs. Robert C. Tarazi and Subha Sen were the first to show reversal of cardiac hypertrophy by various antihypertensive drugs.

8. The Department of Artificial Organs is a legacy from the days of Kolff. His associate Dr. Yukihiko Nosé continued the experimental and developmental work with artificial kidneys and hearts, and when Kolff left, the laboratory returned administratively to the Division of Research (1967), where Nosé is department chairman.

Chapter Nine

1. "Residents" and "fellows" are terms used interchangeably. Because the training programs at the Clinic were called "fellowships" in the early days, the term "fellow" was often used.

2. Dr. William Proudfit recalls, "The entire formal educational experience when I was in training was a weekly lecture for fellows—all the fellows, regardless of specialty. This was held in the evening, and the same program was repeated annually (an advantage, for we learned what lectures to miss!). How that contrasts with the present programs! An internist or a surgeon was expected to be competent in all subspecialties (except, perhaps, allergy for internists and neurosurgery and orthopedics for surgeons)."

3. The charter reads as follows:

Articles of Incorporation of The Frank E. Bunts Educational Institute

The undersigned, all of whom are citizens of the United States, desiring to form a corporation, not for profit, under the General Corporation Act of the State of Ohio, do hereby certify:

First. The name of said corporation shall be The Frank E. Bunts Educational Institute.

Second. The place in said state where the principal office of said corporation shall be located is Cleveland in Cuyahoga County.

Third. The purposes for which said corporation is formed are: to establish, maintain and conduct an institution of learning for promoting education and giving instruction in the art, science and practice of medicine, surgery, anatomy, hygiene and allied or kindred sciences and subjects; to acquire, own, lease, mortgage, pledge, maintain, operate and dispose of real estate, buildings, equipment and other property which may be necessary or useful in connection with promoting education and giving instruction in the sciences and subjects aforesaid; to co-operate with The Cleveland Clinic Foundation, a corporation not for profit organized under the laws of the State of Ohio, and in connection therewith, to make joint or common use of its property and facilities; to accept and receive gifts, bequests and devises of funds, securities and mortgage, pledge, and dispose of funds, securities and property so acquired; and to do any and all things which may be necessary or incident to said purposes.

Fourth. The names and post office addresses of the persons who are to serve as trustees until the first annual meeting or other meeting called to elect trustees are as follows:

Charles F. Thwing, 11109 Bellflower Road,
Cleveland, Ohio;
William E. Wickenden, 11125 Bellflower Road,
Cleveland, Ohio;
Frank A. Quail, 2201 Harcourt Drive,
Cleveland Heights, Ohio;
George Crile, 2620 Derbyshire Road,
Cleveland Heights, Ohio;
William E. Lower, 11957 Carlton Road,
Cleveland, Ohio;
John Sherwin, Jr., 13415 Shaker Boulevard,
Shaker Heights, Ohio;
Edward C. Daoust, 2323 Stillman Road,
Cleveland Heights, Ohio.

Fifth. The persons named in Article "Fourth" are to be the members of said corporation upon organization.

Sixth. Membership in said corporation shall be limited to members of said The Cleveland Clinic Foundation.

Seventh. No person shall be elected a trustee of said Corporation who at the time is not serving as a trustee of said The Cleveland Clinic Foundation.

In Witness Whereof the undersigned have hereunto subscribed their names at Cleveland, Ohio, this 4th day of January, 1935.

> George W. Crile
> John Sherwin, Jr.
> Edward C. Daoust."

4. There was another reason for changing the name, perhaps an even stronger reason for some persons. It had always been Crile's wish that he not be memorialized or named specifically in any way that would set him apart from the other founders.

What was good for Crile might also be good for Bunts, it was said. Also, Dr. Alexander T. Bunts was retiring from the staff, and with his retirement the only remaining descendant of the founders on the professional staff was Dr. George Crile, Jr. Dr. William J. Engel, soon to retire, was the son-in-law of Dr. Lower.

5. In 1982 the *Cleveland Clinic Quarterly* published its fiftieth anniversary issue. The following remarks are summarized from an article by James S. Taylor, M.D., editor, on the history of the *Quarterly.*

In the first year of publication, the *Quarterly* published six original articles and the balance consisted of reprints. Because of the great depression, the *Quarterly* did not appear in 1933 or 1934. On November 28, 1934, the Medical Board met and decided that the *Quarterly* would no longer publish papers that had appeared in other journals.

Some outstanding contributions to the world literature have been published in the *Quarterly*. The *Quarterly* is distributed without charge to physicians and medical libraries throughout the world. In 1982, circulation exceeded 16,000. It is sent to approximately 2600 alumni of The Cleveland Clinic Educational Foundation and to 1000 medical libraries and medical schools. The remainder are sent to other physicians requesting the journal.

The *Cleveland Clinic Quarterly*, a refereed, indexed journal, is an integral part of the educational activities of the Cleveland Clinic and is underwritten solely by The Cleveland Clinic Educational Foundation. The journal is indexed in *Index Medicus, Chemical Abstracts, Biological Abstracts, Current Contents,* and *Nutritional Abstracts*. It is also microfilmed by University Microfilms International.

6. The first chairman of the Faculty Board was Dr. John Beach Hazard, who served from 1956 to 1958. He was succeeded by Leedham, who served from 1958 to 1962. Dr. H. S. Van Ordstrand was appointed in 1963, and Dr. Penn G. Skillern served as chairman from 1964 to January 1973.

In cooperation with Skillern, who was in charge of the internship program initiated in 1957, Zeiter did much to upgrade the quality of postgraduate education and to support the functions of the library and the editorial, art, and photography departments.

INDEX

Adams, Lou, 83
Administrative Board, 41–42
Ahmad, Muzaffar, 80
American College of Surgeons, 6–7
Anderson, John P., 159
Anderson, Robin, 98, 153, 154
Andison, Harry M., 159
Anesthesiology, Department of, 104–105
  Division of, 104–107
Angiotensin, isolation of, 126–127
Annual Professional Review, 62, 157
Antunez, A. R., 112
Arteriography, coronary, Sones' work on, 71–72
Artificial Organs, Department of, 71
Asadorian, Victoria, 116
Association Building Company, 13
Auble, John A., 157

Baldwin, J. F., 16
Ballard, Lester A., Jr., 98
Banting, Frederick G., 161
Barnes, Arthur, 105
Barr, Emmy, 83
Battle, John D., 78, 166
Best, Charles H., 161
Beven, Edwin G., 100
Bill of Sale, 3–4
Biochemistry Laboratory, development of, 119
Blalock, Alfred, 101
Blood Bank, 120
Bloodgood, Joseph C., 16
Board of Governors
  chairmen appointed by, 155
  Division of Research under, 156
  establishment of, 46–47
  Kiser years of 1976 to present, 60–66, 61, 64
  LeFevre years of 1955–1968, 50, 50–54, 51
  Wasmuth years of 1969–1976, 54–60, 56

Board of Trustees
  chairmen of 1956 to present, 52
  Executive Committee of, 40–41
  salary committee of, 155
Booz, Allen and Hamilton, Foundation study by, 43–44
Boutros, Azmy R., 105
Bradley, Charles, 124
Brown, Charles H., 74
Brown, Helen B., 130
Brownlow, William, 27
Bumpus, F. Merlin, 127, 128, 167
Bunts, Alexander T., 29, 94, 135, 148, 171
Bunts, Frank E., 133
  character of, 11–12
  death of, 21, 22, 144
  in Spanish-American War, 5
  medical education of, 1
  World War I work of, 8–9, 9

Cardiology, research progress in, 161
Cardiothoracic Anesthesia, Department of, 106–107
Cavanaugh, Eileen, 106
Chandler, John R., 43
Ciba Award, 131
Clerkships, 136–137
Cleveland Clinic
  aerial view in 1969, 56
  charter of, 14, 16
  disaster of 1929 at, 25–31, 28
  early development of, 13–23
  educational activities of, 133–138
  first building of, 13, 15
  management and growth of, 49–66
  managerial training for, 157
  medical departments of, 67–121
  new 1985 construction for, 64
  opening of, 16
  research activities of, 123–130
  social responsibility of, 57

Cleveland Clinic Building, 1929 disaster at, 25–31, *28*
Cleveland Clinic Educational Foundation, 134
Cleveland Clinic Foundation, 14, 16
 administrative plan of 1947 for, 43–45
 anniversary of 34th year, 153
 during the Depression, 33–36
 purposes of, 17–18
Cleveland Clinic Hospital, opening of, 21, 22
Cleveland Clinic Naval Reserve Unit, 39–40
Cleveland Clinic Pharmacy, 47
Cleveland Clinic Quarterly, 135
 fiftieth anniversary of, 171
Clinical Virology Laboratory, 120
Clough, John D., 77
Codman, Emory A., 147
Collins, E. N., 74
Collins, H. Royer, 95
Collinwood Eldercare Center, aid to, 157
Colorectal Surgery, Department of, 96, 100
Committee on Research Policy and Administration, 47
Compensation Committee, 155, 157
Computerized axial tomography (CAT), 111, 165
Conomy, John P., 76
Cook, Sebastian A., 113
Corcoran, Arthur C., 125, 154
Cori, Carl F., 128
Cori, Gerty T., 128
Coronary Club, 130
Council for High Blood Pressure Research, 130
Crile, George W., 1–2, 41, 170
 and The American College of Surgeons, 6–7
 and Vero Beach crash, 36–37
 character of, 11
 death of, 40, 151
 Foundation President, 37
 in Spanish-American War, 5
 plane crash of, 149–150
 thyroidectomy by, 82–85, 162
 World War I work of, 7–9, *9*
Crile, George, Jr., 40, *50*, 87, *88*, 156, 171
Crile, Mrs. George, 36–37
Cushing, E. F., 10
Cushing, Harvey, 29

Danielsen, Sharon L., 65
Daoust, Edward C., 13, 39, 41, 170
 death of, 42–43
 Foundation President, 38, 40, *41*

Deodhar, Sharad D., 118
deWolfe, Victor G., 80, 153
Diabetic Service, establishment of, 72
Dickinson, C. J., 168
Dickson, James A., 94
Diggs, Lemuel W., 117
Digital subtraction angiography (DSA), 111, 165
Dimethylsulfoxide (DMSO), Clinic use of, 161
Dinner, Melvyn I., 98
Dinsmore, Robert S., 27, 36, 87, *88*, 135
 death of, 162
Disaster of 1929, 25–31, *28*
 account of E. Perry McCullagh, 145–146
 letters in response to, 146–147
 liability for, 148
 rebuilding after, 34–36, *35*
Dittrick, Howard, 135
Division, definition of, 163
Division of Research, Board responsibility for, 47
Dohn, Donald F., 94
Dunning, Charlotte E., 21
Dustan, Harriet P., 128
Dyment, Paul G., 77

Education, Division of, 133–138, *137*
Education Building, 136, *137*
 bequest for, 53
Effler, Donald B., 71, 90, 100, *101*, 129, 160, 163
Endocrinology, Department of, 72
Engel, William J., 40, *50*, 95, 135, 154, 156, 171
Ernstene, A. Carlton, 40, *50*, 68, 154, 156, 159
 Chief of Medicine, 69–70
Esposito, Salvatore J., 98
Esselstyn, Caldwell B., Jr., 85
Estafanous, F. George, 107
Evans, Richard R., 74
Evarts, Charles M., 95
Eversman, John J., 60
Executive Committee, membership of 1947, 43
Executive Committee of Trustees, 152
Executive Health, Section of, 81

Faculty Board, 135–136
Fairfax Foundation, aid to, 157
Farmer, Richard G., 70
Favaloro, René G., *102*, 103

Fazio, Victor W., 100
Fellowship Committee, 135
Ferrario, Carlos, 168
Fiery, Benjamin F., 43
Fischer, Robert J., 63, 156
Fleshler, Bertram, 74
Forest City Hospital, aid to, 156–157
Frank E. Bunts Educational Institute, 134, 135
   incorporation charter of, 169–170
Fricke, Hugo, 16, 123

G-suit, Crile's suggestion for, 150
Galen, Robert S., 118
Gardner, W. James, 40, 41, *50*, 52, 94, 154, 156
Gavan, Thomas L., 118
General Surgery, Department of, 89–90
Getz, Janet Winters, 151
Gifford, Ray W., 79
Gilchrist, Major General, 29
Gilkison, Conrad C., 146
Glasser, Otto, 108–109, *109*, 124
Go, Raymond, 113
Goldblatt, Harry, 96
Gottron, Richard A., 54, 153, 154, 156
Graber, Elizabeth, 85
Graham, Allen, 114–115, 166
Graham, Evarts, 86, 100
Green, Arda, 126, 128
Green, Ralph, 119, 120
Greenhouse, Arnold H., 76
Gross, Robert, 101
Groves, Laurence K., *101*
Gutman, Froncie A., 97
Gynecology, Department of, 97–98

Haden, Russell L., 34, 39, 41, 116–117, 151, 159
   Chief of Medicine, 67–68, *68*
Hahn, Joseph F., 94
Hainline, Adrian, 117
Hale, Donald E., *101*, 104–105, 164
Halle, Walter M., 43, 149
Hamby, Wallace B., 94
Hamilton and Associates, planning report of 1980, 63
Harding, James G., 54, 156
Harris, Harold E., 91
Hart, William R., 119
Hartsock, Charles L., 110, 133, 159
Hartwell, Shattuck W., Jr., 59, 99
Hawk, William A., 117
Hayes, Walter, 121

Hazard, John Beach, *115*, 115–116, 154, 171
Hematology, Department of, 78, 159
Hematology and Medical Oncology, Department of, 159
Hematology Laboratory, 119
Hermann, Robert E., 89
Herrick, Myron T., 7
Hewlett, James S., 78, 166
Higgins, Charles C., 95
Hinnant, I. M., 74
Hoeltge, Gerald A., 120
Hoerr, Stanley O., 98, 154
Hoffman, George C., 118, 166
Holden, Arthur S., Jr., 52
Homi, John, 99
Howe, Charles, 16
Hughes, C. Robert, 109–110, 153
Hughes, James A., 52, *61*, 150
Humphrey, David C., 79
Humphries, Alfred W., 99, 153
Hyatt, Roger C., 30
Hypertension
   Crile's work on, 70
   Department of, 79, 159
   research on, 125–126, 167
Hypertension and Nephrology, Department of, 96, 159

Immunology, Department of, 130
In Memoriam, 148
Infectious Disease, Department of, 80–81
Internal Medicine, Department of, 78–79, 159

Jennings, Martha Holden, 53
John, Henry J., 16, 20, 67, 72, 116
Johnson, William O., 133
Johnston, C. R. K., 74
Jones, John, 101
Jones, Thomas E., 16, 23, 36, 39, 41, 43, 45, 152, 163
   Chief of Surgery, 85–87, *86*
   death of, 87
Jordan, Edwin P., 135

Kaiser Wilhelm Institute, 167
Karch, George, 52
Karnosh, Louis J., 75
Kelley, Joseph F., 74
Kendrick, James I, 94
Kennedy, Roscoe J., 40, 97

Kenneth Clement Family Care Center, aid to, 157
Kidney dialysis program, 79
Kidney transplant program, 96
Kimball, Oliver P., 16, 159
King, John W., 117
Kirklin, John W., 160
Kiser, William S., 47, 58–59, *61*
Kohlstaedt, Helmer, 167
Kohlstaedt, Kenneth, 167
Kolff, Willem J., 71, *101*, 101–102, 128, 160
Krieger, James S., 89, 90, 97–98

Laboratory Medicine, Division of, 114–132, *115*, *119*
Laboratory Medicine Building, *119*
Laurel School, 30
Leedham, Charles L., 135, 171
Lees, James E., 65, 156
LeFevre, Fay A., 49, *50*, *51*, 52, 80, 135, 153, 154, 156
Lewis, Lena A., 124
Livingston, Robert B., 78
Locke, Charles E., Jr., 27, 29, 145
Loop, Floyd D., 103
Lovshin, Leonard L., 59, 79
Lowenthal, Gilbert, Jr., 81
Lower, William E., 41, 170
    medical education of, 5
    personality of, 11
    surgeon to 9th U.S. Cavalry, 5
    World War I work of, 8
Lyman, Sarah E., 30

MacIntyre, W. James, 113
Management Group, establishment of, 60
Marine, David, 116, 166
Marks, Harry T., *61*
Masson, Georges M. C., 128
Master Plan of 1980, 158
Mather, Samuel, 30
Mayo, William J., 16, 114
    Cleveland Clinic opening address of, 19–20
Mayo Clinic, 16, 155, 161
Mayo Foundation, 16
McBride, Edith, 150
McBride, Sarah Tod, 148
McCormack, Lawrence J., 117
McCubbin, James W., 128
McCullagh, E. Perry, 41, *50*, 67, 72, 124, 156
McHenry, Martin C., 81

McLean, Donald H. Jr., 154
Meaney, Thomas F., 110, 135, 168
Medical Survey Committee, 153
    organizational investigation by, 46–47
    recommendations of, 153–154
Medicine, Division of, 67–82
    growth of, 70
Mercer, Robert D., 76, 154
Metabolic Bone Laboratory, 120
Metropolitan Health Planning Corporation, 157
Meyer, E. T., 110
Meyer Medical Magnetic Resonance Center, *111*
Michener, William M., 135
Microbiology, Department of, 120
Mobile Hospital No. 4, 40, 150–151
Molecular and Cellular Biology, Department of, 130
Moore, Paul M., 91
Mullin, William V., 39, 91
Museum of Intelligence, Power and Personality, 148–149

National Diet–Heart Study, 130
National Health Planning and Resources Development Act of 1979, 158
Nelson, Paul A., 78
Netherton, Earl W., 67
Neurological Surgery, Department of, 94
Neurology, Department of, 75–76
Neuropsychiatry, Department of, 75
Nichols, Bernard H., 16, 41, 107–108
Nichols, Don H., 40
Nichols, James H., 54
Nosé, Yukihiko, 168
Nosik, William A., 40
Nuclear magnetic resonance, 111–112
Nursing services, 65

Obstetrical service, closing of, 53
Office of Fund Development, 65
Office of Professional Affairs, 59
Office of Public Affairs, 65–66
Olmsted, Frederick, 129
Orthopedic Surgery, Department of, 94–95
Osborn Building, move to, 5, *7*
Osmond, J. D., 6
Otolaryngology and Communicative Disorders, Department of, 90–93
Oxley, Emma M., 20
Oxley Homes, 20–21, *22*

Packard, Mrs. James, 23
Page, Irvine H., 47, *50*, 52, 124–125, *125*, 154, 156
Pain Therapy Unit, 106
Peart, W. Stanley, 127
Pediatric and Adolescent Medicine, Department of, 159
Pediatric Cardiology, Department of, 159
Pediatrics, Department of, 76–77, 159
Peripheral Vascular Disease, Department of, 80, 159
Section of, 79
Perkins, Litta, 30
Phillips, John, 10, 67, 158
character of, 12
death of, 29
Plan of Organization, August 14, 1947, 44–45
Planning Committee, 46–47, 154
Plastic Surgery, Department of, 92–93, 98
Plummer, Henry, 82, 161.
Portmann, U. V., 23, 108
Portzer, Marietta, 106
Potter, J. Kenneth, 105
Poutasse, Eugene F., 168
Preventive Medicine, Department of, 81
Primary Health Care, Department of, 81
Professional Policy Committee, 46, 152
Professional Staff Affairs, 59
Proudfit, William L., 160, 169
Psychiatry, Department of, 76
Pulmonary Disease, Department of, 80

Quail, Frank A., 170
Quiring, Daniel, 36, 124

Radiology, Division of, 107–114, *109, 111*
Radiotherapy, Department of, 23
Rappaport, Maurice, 126
Reich, Alfred, 116
Renovascular disease, progress in, 96
Resch, Charles A., 99
Research, Division of, 123–132, 156
Research Building, *132*
Research Projects Committee, 47, 127
Rheumatic and Immunologic Disease, Department of, 159
Rheumatic Disease, Department of, 77–78, 159
Rice, Frank A., 146–147
Robnett, Ausey H., 153
Rockefeller, John D. III, 154
Root, Joseph C., 40

Rossmiller, Harold R., 154
Ruedemann, A. D., 27, 39, 41, 97, 151, 163
Ryan, Edward J., 40

Saarel, Douglas A., 60
Scherbel, Arthur L., 77, 154, 161
Schwyzer, Robert, 127
Seitz, Valentine, 23, 108
Selye, Hans, 128
Sen, Subha, 129, 168
Senhauser, Donald A., 118
Serotonin, isolation of, 126
Shafer, William H., 79
Shainoff, John R., 130
Sheldon, William C., 74
Sherman, Henry S., 37, 38, *38*, 39, 41, 150
Sherrer, Edward, 145
Sherwin, John, Jr., 40, 43, 45, 52, 170
Shofner, Nathaniel S., 133
Shupe, Thomas P., 6, 16
Skeggs, Leonard T., 127
Skillern, Penn G., 171
Sloan, Harry G., 6, 8, 16
Sones, F. Mason, Jr., 71, *101, 102*, 129, 160
South Clinic building, 160
Sparks, Irene, 117
Spence, Audrey, 106
Standards Laboratory of the College of American Pathologists, 121
Steinhilber, Richard M., 76
Stewart, Bruce H., 89
Stouffer, Vernon, 131
Stouffer Prize, 131
Straffon, Ralph A., 89, 96
Sullivan, Benjamin H., Jr., 74
Surgery, Division of, 82–104

Tarazi, Robert C., 168
Tautkins, Barney, 113
Taylor, Clarence M., *44*, 44–45, 153
Taylor, James S., 171
Taylor, Robert D., 79, 125
Telkes, Maria, 123
Thomas, J. Warrick, 74
Thoracic and Cardiovascular Surgery, Department of, 53
Thoracic Surgery, Department of, 100
Thwing, Charles F., 21, 170
Thyroidectomy, by George W. Crile, 82–85, 162
Tomashefski, Joseph F., 80
Towers, Perrin, Forster and Crosby, compensation consultation by, 157–158

Transplantation program, 79
Tucker, Harvey M., 93
Tucker, John P., 16, 79, 159
Turnbull, Rupert B. Jr., 87, 100

Urology, Department of, 95–97

Van Ommen, Ray A., 70, 79, 81
Van Ordstrand, H. S., 69, 70, 80, 171
Vascular Surgery, Department of, 99–104, 101
Vero Beach crash, 36–37
Viljoen, John F., 105
Virden, John C., 43

Wasmuth, Carl E., 49, 54–60, 56, 105, 156
Waugh, Justin M., 16, 90

Weatherhead, A. Dixon, 76
Weed, Frank J., 1, 2
  16 Church Street office of, 2
  death of, 2–4
  estate sale of, 3–4
Weick, James K., 78
West Cleveland office, 6
Whitman, John F., 153
Wickenden, William E., 170
Widman, Paul E., 156
Wilde, Alan H., 95
Williams, Guy H., Jr., 40, 75
Willis, Charles E., 118
Wolf, Gerald E., 63, 157
World War I, 7–9, 9

Young, Jess R., 80

Zeiter, Walter J., 50, 135, 153

The text of this book has been set in Palatino. This typeface was designed by Hermann Zapf, one of Europe's greatest contemporary type designers, and it was first produced in 1950 by the Stempel Foundry of Germany. Palatino is named after a historically famous penman of the sixteenth century. Zapf's design is in the tradition of the Venetian family of roman typefaces.

Display Type: Americana
Text Type: Palatino
Book Design: Terri Siegel
Paper: 55 lb. Sebago Antique Offset, S. D. Warren Company, Westbrook, ME
Typography by William J. Dornan, Inc., Collingdale, PA
Manufactured by Maple-Vail Book Manufacturing Group, York, PA